Treatment of AIDS with Traditional Chinese Medicine

Compiler

Zhong DaJin Wang Xuao

Zhao Shuzhen Fu Lining

Revised & translated by

Wang Qiliang

Shandong Science and Technology Press

Editor in Charge : Li Yu

First Edition 1992

Treatment of AIDS with Traditional Chinese Medicine

Compiler Zhong Dajin Wang Xuao Zhao Shuzhen Fu Lining

Revised & translated by Wang Qiliang

Published by Shandong Science and Technology Press

Printed by Foreign Language Printig House

Distributed by China International Book Trading Corporation

35 Chegongzhuang Xilu, Beijing 100044, China

P.O. Box 399, Beijing, China

ISBN7-5331-0993-3/R·249

Printed in the People's Republic of China

FOREWORD

Due to the rapid spread of AIDS all over the world, threatening the health of mankind and the tranquility of human society, various countermeasures have been suggested and executed in most countries. But up to now, none of the pharmacologic agents or vaccines prepared are proved to be satisfactory.

Reports all over the world have shown that TCM is effective in treating AIDS. On basis of relevant informations and our own clinical experiences, we compiled this monograph as a reference to medical Personnel engaged in the prophylaxis and treatment of AIDS.

Compiler

PREFACE

AIDS is an infectious disease with extremely high mortality. It was identified in the beginning of 1980s, and had been called the "supercarcinoma". Shortly after its identification, within several years, AIDS spread all over the world and has become a serious problem. In order to find out effective measures for its prophylaxis and treatment, medical scientists of various countries are engaged in the research of traditional Chinese drugs and traditional Chinese therapies, and they look forward eagerly to new advances in this domain.

Developed and established through thousands of years, TCM is based on unique theoretical systems and rich clinical experiences. It is well known that under TCM therapy, not only common diseases of various departments may be treated successfully, but difficult and complicated cases may also be managed with satisfactory results. Hence, there is a broad prospect of seeking effective measures for the extermination of AIDS through the exploration and investigation of TCM.

Research workers of Treating AIDS with Combined TCM and Western Medicine in Zhejiang Province of China had observed and treated patients infected by HIV for nearly three years. These patients were infected by infusion of imported blood products. Through meticulous and systematic observation of disease conditions and accumulation of clinical experiences, they acquired a new understanding about the cause, pathogenesis, and Syndrome Differentiation and Therapy Selection of AIDS from the viewpoint of TCM. On bases of clinical practice and relevant informations both at home and abroad, they compiled this monograph. It is the first book in China expounding the prophylaxis and treatment of AIDS with TCM, and will certainly contribute to the research in this arduous task.

Violent infectious diseases such as smallpox, plague, cholera, etc., have been conquered by mankind; cancer is being conquered. Beyond doubt, AIDS will be conquered eventually.

He Ren

CONTENTS

Section 1. Brief Recommendation of the Epidemic State of AIDS and Countermeasures against It

During 1979-1980, Pneumocystis carinii pneumonia and Kaposi's sarcoma occurred in a number of male homosexuals in America (Los Angeles, New York, San Francisco, etc.). Later, manifestations of immunodeficiency were also noticed in these patients. At June 1981, CDC for the first time reported a new, independent syndrome through MMWR (Morbidity and Mortality Weekly Report), 5 cases of male homosexuals suffering from Pneumocystis carinii pneumonia were covered. The next month in that year, 26 cases of male homosexuals suffering from Kaposi's sarcoma were reported. Since then, the new, independent morbidity was formally named AIDS (Acquired Immune Deficiency Syndrome).

AIDS is a kind of pernicious infectious disease with a very high mortality, it spreads rapidly all over the world. Medical scientists had demonstrated it is caused by HTLV-III / LAV, or Human T Lymphotropic Retrovirus III / Lymphadenopathy Associated Virus, because characteristics of this disease are the loss of selective activity of T helper lymphocytes and the serious damage of immunologic mechanism.

At June 1986, International Nomenclature Committee for Virus of AIDS suggested to replace HTLV-III, LAV, ARV (AIDS Associated Retrovirus) by HIV (Human Immunodeficiency Virus).

However, a second type (HIV-2) was separated from AIDS patients by American and English researchers. Such virus was found in certain districts of Western Africa, but it is rare in high risk populations of other continents. At the 4th International Meeting on AIDS, Belgian medical workers claimed the existence of HIV-3, but there was no consensus. Jean Claude, the director of Retrovirus Laboratory, Marseilles, France, had pointed out: Only when a virus cannot be detected by current laboratory technique, could a new virus naming be granted. Moreover, such virus should be isolated from AIDS patients, whose serum must be negative in both HIV-1 and HIV-2.

I. Brief Survey of the Epidemic State of AIDS all over the World

It is said that originally AIDS occurred in Zaire, Africa. Thereafter it spreads swiftly from Zaire to America and Western Europe, then all over the world. The quick transmission of this disease may be illustrated by the following data:

In 1981, the first case of AIDS was formally reported in America.

In December 1982, a total of 711 cases in 16 countries was reported.

On 14th November, 1986, 34 443 cases in 77 countries had been reported to WHO Global Control Programme of AIDS.

On 1st April, 1987, 45 700 cases in 131 countries and districts had been reported to WHO.

In July 1987, there were 55 396 AIDS patients in 142 countries and districts.

On 12th January, 1988, 75 392 cases of AIDS were reported.

Officials of WHO hold, the actual number of AIDS patients would be at least twice as those reported by various countries, owing to the lack of relevant knowledge and missing of reports. At present, it is estimated that the total number of patients infected by HIV all over the world amounts to 5-10 million. Therefore, AIDS will spread even more widely and seriously, unless it is controlled or exterminated.

The number of AIDS cases in America accounts for 68.8% of the whole world; the mortality is as high as 85%. Now, 1.2-1.5 million people are infected by HIV; among them, 10-20% are patients with symptoms and signs of AIDS. The American Ministry of Health has predicted that the number of AIDS patients will reach 270 000 in 1991. In addition, the number of people infected by HIV and patients suffering from AIDS is increasing rapidly in Europe, Asia, Oceania, and Africa.

On 25th February, 1989, a monitoring result covering 70 000 people was reported in PRC; 22 people with HIV antibody and 3 patients suffering from AIDS were detected. Among them, 4 are Chinese, caused by infusion of imported Factor VIII; the rest are foreigners or foreign citizens of Chinese origin.

As to routes, modes, and epidemic style of AIDS transmission, there has been a comparatively clear understanding on the basis of epidemiologic investigation.

I) Routes of AIDS transmission

There are three routes of AIDS transmission: Sexual contact, infusion of blood products, and diaplacental infection.

II) Factors related to AIDS transmission

1. Male homosexuality with many sexual partners (accounts to 70-80%), and males indulging in heterosexuality.
2. Abuse of addictive drugs administered intravenously, such

as heroine, cocaine, etc., in the past or at present.

3. Hemophiliacs or patients who need frequent blood transfusion.
4. Infants born by mothers suffering from AIDS. The infection rate comes up to 70%.
5. Immigration. 4% immigrants from Haiti are AIDS sufferers.

III) Modes of AIDS transmission

1. Sexual derangement. There are a large amount of virus and lymphocytes in the semen of AIDS patient. During sexual intercourse, HIV may pass through damaged mucous membrane and infect the partner.
2. Infusion of HIV-infected blood or blood products, especially concentrated Factor VIII, because it is generally a mixed preparation collected from 2 000 to 20 000 people.
3. Injured skin exposed to HIV, or the use of HIV-contaminated syringe or syringe needle.
4. Perinatal infection.

IV) Epidemic styles of AIDS

Epidemiologic investigations had revealed that the epidemic styles of AIDS in various continents are different. Their characteristics are as follows:

1. The first style

The epidemic style of AIDS in America, Western Europe, and Oceania is characterized by the typical "Western" style described by American medical workers first. In other words, it is transmitted mainly through male homosexuality, heterosexuality, or intravenous injection of addictive drugs. Other transmissive routes constitute only a small percentage.

2. The second style

The epidemic style of AIDS in Africa is somewhat different from that of the typical "Western" one. It is transmitted mainly through heterosexual intercourse (male AIDS infects female partner or female AIDS infects male partner), blood transfusion, or HIV-contaminated syringe or syringe needle.

3. The third style

The epidemic style of AIDS in Asia, Eastern Europe, and the Pacific district is characterized by infusion of imported blood products or by sexual transmission through prostitutes.

The quick spread of AIDS throughout the whole world exerts a tremendous influence over human society. The prognosis of AIDS is ominous. Moreover, asymptomatic HIV carriers are subjected to extraordinary mental pressure, because their kinsfolk and friends are afraid to keep in contact with them. Fear of being infected and the doom of parents disintegrate the family. Falling ill and the decrease of productive population bring about huge economic losses in developed and developing countries. In Africa, the mortality of children rises sharply. Therefore, enormous human, financial, and material resources have been thrown into the research of its prophylaxis and treatment. Consequently, current system of health care, insurance, legal provisions, etc., will be deeply influenced too.

II. Countermeasures for the Prophylaxis and Treatment of AIDS

Up to now it is evident that no country or district can escape the invasion of AIDS, and no country or district can deal with this disease independently. Extensive international cooperation and joint action are absolutely necessary. Several years ago, 12 concrete demands had been proposed by WHO, which should be carried out by health departments of various countries to prevent the transmission of AIDS. Among them, there are publicity and education, training of medical personnel, establishment of monitoring organizations, strict control of blood products, timely presenting reports about the epidemic state of AIDS to WHO, etc.Owing to the rapid variation of HIV, effective vaccine against AIDS has not been prepared successfully.

According to results of current research, principal countermeasures are as follows:

I) Prophylactic measures

1. Wide-spread publicity and education

In view of the fact that effective vaccines are not available at present, the crux of AIDS prophylaxis lies chiefly in the publicity and education of the masses. These are aimed at:

1) Explaining the epidemic style of AIDS and the route of its transmission, thereby to refrain the masses from sexual derangement and / or visiting prostitutes, so as to protect themselves well.

2) Eliminating the terror-stricken frame of mind of the public, relieving the social isolated state and mental solitariness of AIDS patients, encouraging them to fight against the disease.

2. Prevention of hematogenous transmission

1) Establish laboratories for detecting HIV antibody in blood samples taken from blood donors; stop the use of blood, blood products, organs, semen, and other tissues with HIV antibody or those contaminated by HIV.

2) Pregnancy should be contraindicated in female AIDS patients or females with HIV antibody.

3) Forbid the abuse of intravenous injection to reduce the danger of AIDS transmission; advocate to use syringe and its needle only for once.

3. Sterilization

HIV may be inactivated by ordinary disinfectants, detergents, or at 56°C for 30 min. It cannot survive in a dry environment.

Contaminated objects may be disinfected by cleansing them with freshly prepared 500-5 000 ppm sodium hypochlorite solution (diluted 1:10-100) or by boiling them under certain circumstances. 1:10 diluted bleaching powder may be used in home disinfection. Besides, 5% formalhyde, 2% glutaraldehyde, or 70% alcohol are also effective.

4. Preparation of AIDS vaccine

Vaccination is the most effective measure to control epidemic disease. Unfortunately up to now, no success has been obtained in the preparation of effective vaccine for preventing AIDS. Nevertheless, scientific researchers have not been disappointed of their purpose; failure is the mother of success.

5. Reinforcement of sanitary surveillance and legislation

Since the perniciousness and seriousness of AIDS had been recognized, stern measures were adopted by many countries and districts. Prostitutes, prisoners, drug addicts, and patients suspected to be suffering from AIDS are examined compulsorily, pregnant women are included also. In addition, Centres for AIDS Prevention or similar organizations have been established generally. In some of these Centres, screening of blood donors is carried out as a routine task. Legal provisions for preventing AIDS are under discussion in Japan.

So far AIDS patients discovered in China are foreign tourists and those who received imported blood products. Under these circumstances, China Ministry of Health and the Head Office of

Customs had notified that the importation of blood products should be stopped. As to those already imported, strict quarantine should be carried out. AIDS had been rated as an infectious disease of B class in 1986. A coordinative group for its monitoring has been organized by Chinese Centre of Preventive Medicine.

II) Therapeutic measures

1. Anti-HIV drugs

Medical scientists in various countries are working hard and perseveringly to search for drugs that may prevent HIV infection and inhibit the replication of HIV. Many drugs have been tried clinically, but their effects are not satisfactory. Here, some of them are recommended as follows:

1) Suramin sodium

This is a blocking agent of reverse transcriptase (RT). In vitro, it may almost completely inhibit the replication of HIV and prevent its infection. De Clercq reported in 1977 that this drug may inhibit the activity of RT of retrovirus in animals. Clinically, complete inhibition of HIV was achieved by the administration of 0.2g / ml suramin sodium accompanied with side-effects, such as fever, acute neurotic disturbance, anaphylaxis, abnormality of hepatic function, etc. Yet no toxic reactions occurred when 7 cases of early AIDS were treated with this drug (2g / week) for 6 weeks.

2) Azidothymidine (AZT)

AZT is the first drug approved by FDA (Food and Drug Adiministration, USA) for treating AIDS experimentally. It can inhibit the activity of RT, suppress the synthesis of proteinic core of HIV, and permeate into CNS through the BBB. AZT can be taken orally. 200 cases of AIDS had been treated with this drug since 1986. According to one report, among 148 cases of AIDS taking AZT, only one patient died. Meanwhile among 131 cases taking placebo, sixteen died. After the administration of AZT, body weight and the amount of T lymphocyte were increased. Main toxic effects of this drug is the inhibition of hemopoietic function of bone marrow, leading to anemia and leukopenia.

3) Antimony tungstate (HPA-23)

Antimony tungstate may inhibit the replication of virus and lead to thrombocytopenia. 50 cases of early, advanced AIDS, and AIDS with complications were treated with this drug in Paris; 80 cases of AIDS were treated with this drug in America. Therapeutic effects have not been evaluated yet.

4) Foscarmet sodium

This drug is used in Sweden as an anti-herpes agent; it may destroy the proteinic capsule of virus. In vitro, results of experiments have shown that the RT of HIV is inhibited very efficiently by low concentration of foscarmet sodium.

5) α-Interferon

This drug inhibits the replication of HIV. But unlike ordinary cytotoxic drugs, it does not impair the debilitated immunologic system of AIDS patients further. Thus the danger of casual infection may be reduced which is often fatal. Krown, et al. reported that 7 among 12 cases of AIDS survived after the intramuscular administration of recombinative α-interferon. Chief side-effects were influenza-like syndrome accompanied with fever, headache, and indisposition, inhibition of bone marrow, and reversible elevation of transaminase level.

6) Glycyrrhizin

Japanese scholar Itonasayuki demonstrated in 1987 that this drug may inhibit the replication of HIV. (2 cases of AIDS, 2 cases of ARC, and 7 cases of HIV carrier were treated with neominophagen C, which contains 40 mg of glycyrrhizin. 8 weeks later, the ratio of CD_4/CD_8 rises in 6 cases among 7 HIV carriers. Moreover, the number of CD_4 cells increases in 4 patients. But these improvements do not occur in patients suffering from AIDS and ARC.

2. Traditional Chinese Medicine

It is common knowledge that TCM is a great treasure-house. Since the first case of AIDS was reported in America, foreign medical workers become enthusiastic about the application of TCM in AIDS prophylaxis and treatment. Relevant explorations and researches have been conducted and encouraging therapeutic results have been obtained. For instance, in addition to traditional Chinese medicinal herbs and prescriptions, acupuncture-moxibustion and Qigong are found to be effective in alleviating symptoms and signs of AIDS, such as debility, fatigability, shortness of breath, night sweat, diarrhea, lymphadenectasis, pain, numbness, etc.

Therefore, boundless prospects of treating AIDS with combined TCM and current medicine are spreading out before us, if they are incorporated correctly and skillfully.

Section 2. Etiology and Pathogenesis of AIDS from the Viewpoint of TCM

I. Characteristics of the Rationale of TCM

I) The concept of holism

According to TCM, there is a correspondence between mankind and the universe; in other words, there are corresponding relations between the anatomical structures, physiological functions, and pathological changes of human body and the natural environment.

II) Causes of disease and pathogenesis

From the viewpoint of TCM, all factors and conditions which destroy physiologic equilibrium and bring about functional imbalance or disturbance are causes of disease. They are divided into endopathogens, exopathogens, and non-endo-non-exo-pathogens. As to pathogenesis, there are the famous Nineteen Items of Pathogenesis defined in *Familiar Conversation*. It is natural that concepts of causes and pathogenesis are similar in Western medicine and TCM, but they are not identical, there are many differences in their connotations.

III) Pathogenic Evil and Healthy Energy

Ancient doctors had pointed out in *Familiar Conversation* that whenever the body is attacked by Evils, there must be

Asthenia of Healthy Energy. In a morbid state, Pathogenic Evil is on one side, Healthy Energy or body resistance is on the other side. Therefore, disease condition may be regarded as the manifestation of the wrestling state between Pathogenic Evil and Healthy Energy.

IV) Evidence Differentiation and Therapy Selection

External manifestations of a morbid state is called Evidence or Syndrome in TCM. Since there are differences in natural environment and differences in mental, physical, and nutritional states, various symptoms and signs may occur when people are attacked by the same Pathogenic Evil. It is also evident that in different stages of the same disease, clinical manifestations are different. Therefore, patients should be treated individually according to his (her) concrete condition.

II. Pathogenesis of AIDS from the Viewpoint of TCM

There are no records or descriptions about AIDS in TCM. Although in the early stage of AIDS manifestations of virus infection may occur and it seems appropriate to treat it by adopting the diagnostic and therapeutic methods proposed in *Treatise on Pestilence* (Wu Youxing, 1642), but soon afterwards, its development is quite different from that of pestilence. Asthenic Syndrome occurs constantly and runs through the whole course of AIDS.

I) Significance of Healthy Energy depletion in AIDS

Epidemiologic investigation had revealed that AIDS generally occurs in homosexual males and drug addicts abusing intravenous injection. Homosexual males are sexually paranoiac and extremely fervent in libido. Their frequency of sexual intercourse far exceeds that of normal men. TCM holds: "Kidney is the origin of congenital constitution and it is responsible for the storation of semen or Essence of Life". Indulgence in libido inevitably depletes Kidney Essence and debilitates Healthy Energy. Yu Jinghe, a famous physician in Qing Dynasty had pointed out: "Females belong to Yin. Yin is adept in lying and streaming downwards. Males belong to Yang. Sexual intercourse between two men signifies the combination of two Yang. Since there is no way to discharge the Ministerial Fire, Flaming Toxin accumulates in the rectum and invades his partner through the penis". According to this account, homosexuality between two men not only depletes their Kidney Essences, but also brings about the danger of Flaming Toxin invasion.

Drug addicts constitute another group of people susceptible to AIDS. Heroin, cocaine, marijuana, opium preparations, etc. are addictive drugs. It had been pointed out that all pungent-hot natured drugs damage Essence and Yin and opium is the most pungent-hot one (*Impart Knowledge of Consumptive Diseases by Heart*). Wang Yu (Qing Dynasty) in *Medical Records beside the Drunken Flower Window* stressed: "Opium is the most fierce drug in drying Lung Energy. Indulgence of taking opium leads to dryness of Qi and Blood". Similar viewpoints had also been declared in other medical books, such as *Deserted House Medical Talks*. Therefore, the harmfulness of addictive drugs is also well-known in China.

To sum up, homosexuality and drug addiction provide a basis for HIV infection, and the HIV infection further impairs one's Healthy Energy. Thus we hold, Asthenia is the principal aspect or feature of AIDS.

II) Significance of Pathogenic Evil in the onset of AIDS

In TCM, there are only wordings of "Pestilent toxin", "Epidemic evil", "Fierce filth", etc. , which represent different kinds of pathogenic factors. Nevertheless, HIV may also be regarded as the pathogenic evil of AIDS from the viewpoint of TCM.

Whatever the pathogenic factor may be, after it has invaded human body, the condition of Healthy Energy plays an important role in deciding whether there will be an onset of disease or not. If the Healthy Energy is exuberant or the pathogenic factor is comparatively weak, there will be no onset of disease or the onset is slow and mild. If the Healthy Energy is debilitated or the pathogenic factor is comparatively ferocious, there will be a prompt onset of disease with a serious outcome. Obviously the invasion of a pathogenic factor itself does not inevitably cause an onset. These may explain the following fact: Among the people having been infected by HIV under similar circumstances, only a small part of them become AIDS patients, while most of them remain chronic HIV carriers.

According to TCM, "Dominance of Evils leads to Sthenia"; "Depletion of Healthy Energy leads to Asthenia". The relation between Asthenia and Sthenia may be very intricate. Sometimes Sthenia is complicated by Asthenia; sometimes Asthenia is complicated by Sthenia.

In short, the most outstanding feature or problem of AIDS is the serious damage of human immunologic function, which may be regarded as the depletion or debility of Healthy Energy from our viewpoint. Moreover, data of current pharmacologic studies have also demonstrated that the strengthening of Healthy Energy is featured by the improvement or the regulation of immunologic function. Inspired by these findings, we believe the application of TCM in treating AIDS is bound to be a success.

Section 3. Chief Clinical Manifestations of AIDS and Their Evidence Differentiation according to TCM

I. Chief Clinical Manifestations of AIDS

AIDS usually occurs in young and middle-aged people, mostly (90%) between 20-49 years of age. AIDS patients below 20 years of age or over 60 are rarely encountered. The ratio of morbidity between males and females is 14:1.

The latent period of AIDS (from HIV infection to the appearance of clinical manifestation) has not been assessed accurately through direct observation. But according to data accumulated in research of AIDS caused by blood transfusion, it is estimated to be around 29 months in adults, 19.4 months in children. In homosexuals, it is about 38 months. By using a mathematical model, American CDC had calculated the latent period of AIDS and found it to be 1-14 years, on average, 6 years.

Clinically, people infected by HIV may be divided into four types:

I) Asymptomatic HIV carrier

Having been infected by HIV, most people remain virus carriers. According to certain reports, the morbidity of AIDS within 4 years reaches 35%. Generally, no symptoms and signs occur in HIV carriers. But occasionally, there mayb e fatigability and liability of sweating. The following changes may be detected by laboratory examination: Moderate, persistent decrease of the amount of T_4, decline of the T_4/T_8 ratio, positive results of the enzyme-linked immunosorbent assay (ELISA). Moreover, in 50-80% of these people, HIV may be identified.

In these people, there may be no distinct change in the tongue proper, tongue coating, and pulse condition; or there may be pale red tongue, nearly reddened tongue with white and thin coating or greasy and thin coating. The pulse condition may be thready or thready and rapid. These correspond to manifestations of Qi Asthenia or Asthenia of both Qi and Blood.

II) Acute HIV infection

There may be manifestations of fever, chills, headache, arthralgia, lymphadenectasis, even symptoms and signs of aseptic meningitis after 2-4 weeks of HIV infection, resembling those of "viral syndrome", or "monocytosis". Positive ELISA may be detected only within 1-3 months after this acute stage generally.

In this type, there are reddened or crimson tongue with yellow, thin or greasy coating; thready, rapid or bow-string, rapid pulse. These correspond to manifestations of syndromes of Defence, Energy, or Nutrient System in "Epidemic Febrile Disease".

III) AIDS-Related Complex (ARC)

Typical casual infections occur within 1 year in most of these patients. Common symptoms and signs are diarrhea, feebleness, arthralgia, intermittent fever, emaciation, persistent and generalized lymphadencetasis. The latter is especially prominent in areas of the neck and abdomen.

The colour of the tongue proper is usually inclined to pallor, or petechiae or ecchymoses emerge. The tongue coating is yellow or yellow and greasy. The pulse condition is deep and thready, or thready and uneven. These correspond to manifestations of depletion of Healthy Energy, or Phlegm agglutination and Blood stasis.

IV) AIDS

AIDS is characterized by progressive exhaustion of the whole body, loss of body weight, extreme feebleness, and remarkable diarrhea. Data of laboratory examination reveal: Extremely lowered immunocompetence, persistent decrease of T_4, and $T_4/T_8 < 0.5$. Typical casual infections often occur simultaneously, such as Pneumocystis carinii pneumonia, Kaposi's sarcoma, and other malignancies, which are the most commonly encountered.

In this type, generally the tongue proper is pale, the tongue coating is greasy or yellow and greasy. The pulse condition is deep, thready, and feeble. These correspond to Asthenia of Healthy Energy or Asthenia complicated by Sthenia.

II. Evidence Differentiation of AIDS

Although guiding principles and theories are basically the same, various types of Evidence Differentiation of AIDS had been proposed by doctors both in China and in other countries. Some of them hold AIDS should be distinguished into: Depletion of Kidney Yin, Insufficiency of Lung Yin, Blood Activation due to Exuberance of Heat, and Stagnation-Stasis due to Asthenia of Healthy Energy. Later, these had been summed up by other doctors as two categories: Depletion of Lung-Kidney

Yin, and Sinking of Heat into Nutrient-Blood System.

According to our understanding of the pathogenesis and principal aspects of AIDS, we deem it will be better to distinguish AIDS into 10 categories, i.e. Asthenia of both Qi and Yin, Depletion of Qi and Blood, Asthenia and Weakness of Spleen-Stomach, Asthenia of Liver-Kidney Yin, Asthenia of Lung-Kidney Yin, Depression and Stagnation of Liver Qi, Internal Accumulation of Wetness-Turbidity, Blazing of Heat-Toxin, Lucid Aperture Covered by Phlegm, and Phlegm Aggiutination and Blood Stasis.

Section 4. Therapeutic Principles and Chief Methods of TCM in Treating AIDS

According to TCM, relative equilibrium of Yin-Yang is the basis of normal physiological activities of human body. Whenever imbalance of Yin-Yang occurs, there will be illness. Ancient doctors had told us in Chapter 74 of *Familiar Conversation* that medical workers should examine Yin and Yang carefully and regulate them with the aim of restoring their balance. Evidently, Yin-Yang theory is the guide-line of TCM.

Since depletion of Healthy Energy provides the basis for HIV invasion and HIV invasion further depletes Healthy Energy, we hold that AIDS should be treated under the principle of "Strengthening Healthy Energy and Eliminating Pathogenic Evil".

I. Therapeutic Principle of TCM in Treating AIDS

In TCM, there are rich connotations in the principle of "Strengthening Healthy Energy and Eliminating Pathogenic Evil". It may signify "Strengthening Healthy Energy thereby to Eliminate Pathogenic Evil", or "Strengthening Healthy Energy and Eliminating Pathogenic Evil concurrently", or "Eliminating Pathogenic Evil thereby to support Healthy Energy". Therefore, under this principle a variety of therapeutic measures may be selected or combined in the treatment of AIDS.

Ancient doctors had warned us that "While strengthening

Healthy Energy, Pathogenic Evil should not be retained; while eliminating Pathogenic Evil, Healthy Energy should not be harmed". In various stages of AIDS, sometimes we lay stress on the former, sometimes we lay stress on the latter.

In TCM, Strengthening Healthy Energy is also called Strengthening Body Resistance and Consolidating Bodily Foundation. Such measures are aimed at keeping the dynamic equilibrium of Yin and Yang, Solid Viscera and Hollow Viscera, Qi and Blood, etc., thereby to invigorate body resistance and provide material basis for fighting against Pathogenic Evils.

From the viewpoint of TCM, bodily foundation indicates Solid Viscera in the main, especially Kidney, Spleen, and Lung; because "Kidney is the origin of congenital constitution and the reservoir of Visceral Essence and Qi; Spleen provides material basis for the acquired constitution, it is the source of Qi and Blood; Lung is in charge of Qi, Exterior, and Defence System".

"Eliminating Pathogenic Evil" implies the elimination of HIV in current medicine. Through incessant replication, HIV impairs human immunologic function continuously. Therefore, the principle of Eliminating Pathogenic Evil should be observed throughout the entire course of AIDS, and therapeutic measures, regardless of Current and Traditional Chinese Medicine, should be incorporated.

II. Chief Methods of TCM in Treating AIDS

Habitually, therapeutic methods of TCM are classified as Eight Methods: Diaphoresis, emesis, purgation, mediation, warming, heat-reducing, tonification, and elimination. In treating AIDS, tonification, heat-reducing, elimination, and purgation are used more frequently. Specifically speaking, they are methods of tonifying-benefiting, clearing Heat away, activating Blood and resolving stasis, and purging bowels.

I) Method of tonifying-benefiting

According to theories of TCM, "Asthenia should be treated with tonifying therapy". Chinese medicinal herbs with tonifying and benefiting properties are those which may replenish the deficiency or depletion of Yin, Yang, Qi, Blood, Essence, Fluids, etc., and those which may relieve symptoms and signs of Asthenia.

Current pharmacologic studies have demonstrated that these Chinese medicinal herbs may improve debilitated or restore disordered neurohumoral regulatory function, support or reinforce body resistance, and promote or ameliorate functional and structural convalescence.

Chinese medicinal herbs with tonifying and benefiting properties may be distinguished into four kinds:

1. Qi invigorating medicinal herbs
   These include Radix Ginseng, Radix Codonopsis Pilosulae, Radix Astragali seu Hedysari, etc.
2. Blood nourishing medicinal herbs
   These include Radix Angelicae Sinensis, Radix Paeoniae Alba, Radix Rehmanniae, etc.
3. Yin nourishing medicinal herbs
   These include Radix Polygoni Multiflori, Fructus Lycii, Fructus Ligustri Lucidi, etc.
4. Yang invigorating medicinal herbs
   These include Herba Epimedii, Semen Cuscutae, Cordyceps, Sinensis etc.

There are rich proteins, fats, carbohydrates, vitamins, salts, and trace elements essential to human body in tonifying and benefiting medicinal herbs.

It has also been proved that these medicinal herbs may improve immunologic function. For example, animal experiments have shown tonifying and benefiting medicinal herbs may evidently activate the phagocytic function of reticuloendothelial system, influence specific and non-specific immunity, as well as humoral and cellular immunity. Some Chinese medicinal harbs, such as Radix Ginseng, Fructus Ligustri Lucidi, Radix Astragali seu Hedysari, etc., may promote the proliferation of lymphocytes in normal people, bringing about an immunoregulatory effect. Besides, the defensive power against the invasion of foreign bodies is remarkably strengthened in mice by the administration of Radix Acanthopanacis Senticosi.

It has been concluded that Qi invigorating drugs may improve non-specific immunity; Blood nourishing drugs may enrich the blood and regulate cardiovascular system; Yin nourishing drugs may inhibit the hyperactivity of immunologic function, thereby alleviate side-effects caused by the administration of immunosuppressants; Yang invigorating drugs may promote the production of antibody.

Chinese medicinal herbs with tonifying and benefiting properties are of great importance to the prophylaxis and treatment of AIDS because they may safeguard immunologic function and prevent casual infection.

II) Method of clearing away Heat

This is also called the method of clearing away Heat and resolving Toxin. Through the use of drugs which are cool or cold in nature, evil Heat is cleared away and flaming Toxin is resolved. In TCM, more than 1 000 kinds of drugs are cool or cold in nature; among them, about 100 kinds are antibacterials, about 250 kinds are antivirotics. Moreover, these medicinal herbs may influence and improve immunologic function extensively. Thus, they are not only antibacterials and antivirotics, but also immunoregulators.

When Heat-Toxin occurs in AIDS, it should be treated by this method.

III) Method of activating Blood and resolving Stasis

Current pharmacologic researches have demonstrated that Chinese medicinal herbs of activating Blood and resolving Stasis may also eliminate Pathogenic Evils, because they may raise the level of antibody and complement, invigorate immunity, promote the transformation of lymphocytes and the synthesis of DNA and RNA, and regulate the equilibrium of T helper cells and T suppressor cells.

In addition, these kinds of Chinese medicinal herbs may improve blood circulation, especially the microcirculation, facilitating the convalescence of pathologic changes. They may ameliorate capillary permeability, invigorate phagocytic function of phagocytes, mitigate inflammatory reaction, and accelerate its extinction. Besides, they may inhibit the metabolism of connective tissue, promoting its softening and absorption. According to certain reports, they may block the implantation of tumour cells, enhance the sensitivity of chemotherapy, and prevent tissue fibrosis resulted from radiotherapy.

Immunoregulatory, antineoplastic effects and the action of softening and resolving Masses are of great importance in the prophylaxis and treatment of AIDS.

IV) Method of purging

This is also called the method of "Opening the Interior by

Offensive Purging" and held as an important means for eliminating Pathogenic Evils. Wu Youxing had stressed such a viewpoint in his *Treatise on Pestilence*: "The important thing is to drive out exogenous evils early. Because at this moment, patients' Qi and Blood have not been disturbed, body fluids have not been depleted, muscles have not been emaciated. Early driving out of pathogenic evils will not go so far as to endanger the patient. Hence, the composing of prescription will not be restricted, and the convalescence will be easy and smooth". Generally, this method is used to treat Interior-Sthenia-Heat Syndrome. While Evil-Toxin threatens life, even if body fluids are consumed by Heat or protracted illness, this method is not contraindicated.

During certain stages of AIDS, there may be manifestations of Heat Syndrome accompanied with depletion of Yin or body fluids. Under these conditions, the method of purging warrants our consideration.

It is common knowledge that Radix et Rhizoma Rhei is an important ingredient of purging prescriptions. Current pharmacologic studies have revealed that in addition to purging bowels, it may also resist bacterial invasion and tumorigenesis, reduce fever, and stop hemorrhage.

III. Tentative Ideas and Suggestions

Along with the deep-going research of the combination of Western medicine and TCM, the following tentative ideas and suggestions deserve speculation.

I) Seeking for ingredients which may resist HIV infection from Chinese medicinal herbs, including Chinese natural foods

It had been demonstrated that about 250 kinds of Chinese medicinal herbs are antivirotics. Experiments carried out in cultured cells, chicken embryos, and animals in vivo have shown that more than 20 kinds of animal viruses are inhibited by these medicinal herbs, and these drugs are comparatively energetic. Therefore, it is reasonable to hope effective monomers will be refined.

II) Seeking for effective Chinese medicinal herbs or prescriptions which may improve immunologic function

Since Chinese medicinal herbs with tonifying-benefiting properties, with clearing away Heat and detoxifying properties, and with activating Blood and resolving Stasis properties may safeguard immune system and ameliorate immunologic state, we hold that better therapeutic results will be obtained by selecting appropriate drugs to compose new prescriptions.

In fact, it had been demonstrated repeatedly that ginsenosides of Radix Ginseng and polysaccharides of Polyporus Umbellatus may improve immunologic function; saponins contained in Radix Bupleuri Decoction and Radix Ginseng Decoction may activate immunologic function.

III) Improving the therapeutic effect of AIDS by combining TCM with Western medicine

Both TCM and Western medicine are great treasures of mankind; each has its own strong points, and each has its own shortcomings. It goes without saying that by combining their strong points better therapeutic effect would be obtained.

Recently, an American suffering from AIDS was detected in Beijing. Having been diagnosed correctly by scientific techniques, he was treated with TCM measures. Thereafter his symptoms and signs were alleviated and his life-span was lengthened.

IV) Mutual supplementary administration of Western drugs and Chinese medicinal herbs

Simultaneous administration of Western drugs and Chinese medicinal herbs will bring their virtues into full play and overcome their defects. For instance, side-effects such as serious inhibition of hematopoiesis caused by AZT may be alleviated by concurrent administration of Chinese medicinal herbs. On the other hand, effects of Chinese drugs will be strengthened by concurrent administration of Western drugs.

Section 5. Treatment of AIDS in Line with TCM

I. Syndrome Differentiation and Therapy Selection

Under the guidance of unique theories and methodologies of TCM, diseases are treated effectively. It is self evident that a proper treatment comes from a correct diagnosis. In Evidence differentiation or in making a diagnosis, which is the primary cause of the disease and which is the secondary one, which is the Root and which is the Branch, which is of greater urgency and which is of lesser urgency, etc. should be distinguished carefully. The distribution, nature, and the pathogenesis of disease should be ascertained accurately. On such bases, the therapeutic principle is determined and relevant prescription or measure is selected. A feature of TCM is that it often does not regard a kind of disease (from the viewpoint of Western medicine) as a single entity, and treat it with one measure from the beginning to the end, but select different prescriptions or measures in accordance with the variation of disease condition, or the result of Evidence differentiation at the moment.

There are different stages of AIDS with various symptoms and signs. Its disease condition is very changeable and intricate. In order to make it concise, taking Asthenia-Sthenia as the key link of Evidence differentiation, we divide manifestations of AIDS into 10 types. It should be pointed out that clinically, typical and simple Evidence types are seldom encountered.

These 10 types cited below may occur separately and singularly, or two or three of them may occur simultaneously. There may be dominance of Asthenia or a state of mixed Asthenia and Sthenia. Thus, concrete measures should be flexible.

I) Asthenia Syndrome

1. Asthenia of both Qi and Yin

1) Principal symptoms and signs

Listlessness, feebleness, emaciation, shortness of breath, hectic fever, night sweat, dryness of the mouth and throat, dry cough with little sputum; pale red tongue with white and thin coating; thready and weak pulse.

These are commonly encountered in patients infected by HIV, or in patients suffering from ARC.

2) Pathogenesis

Listlessness, feebleness, shortness of breath, etc., are manifestations of Qi Asthenia; hectic fever is caused by Yin Asthenia; dry mouth and throat are due to the deficiency of body fluids; dry cough is due to the failure of moistening action.

3) Therapeutic principle

Invigorate Qi, nourish Yin.

4) Therapy

Chinese medicinal herbs

① Referential prescription

Radix Astragali seu Hedysari Drink for Restoring Pulse Beat.

② Chinese medicinal herbs commonly used

Radix Astragali seu Hedysari (praeparata), Radix Codonopsis Pilosulae (fried), Radix Ophiopogonis, Fructus Schisandrae, Rhizoma Anemarrhenae, Cortex Lycii Radicis, Radix Asparagi.

Formulated preparation: Radix Astragali seu Hedysari Drink for Restoring pulse Beat, 1 ampoule (10 ml), po, bid. Hedysari Drink for Restoring Pulse Beat, 1 ampoule (10 ml), po, bid.

③ Modification of herbs

Dominance of hectic fever: add Radix Gentianae Macrophyllae, Radix Cynanchi Atrati, Radix Stellariae.

Remarkable night sweat: add Concha Ostreae, Fructus Tritici Levis, Radix Oryzae Glutinosae.

Serious dry cough: add Radix Glehniae, Rhizoma Polygonati Odorati, Radix Trichosanthis.

Obvious dryness of the mouth and throat: add Radix Scrophulariae, Herba Dendrobii.

Acupuncture and moxibustion

① Meridians and acupoints commonly selected

SP6 and KI3; adjunct points: ST36, LU9, BL13; invigorating manipulation.

② Modification of acupoints

Cough: add LU5; Hectic fever: add LU10; Night sweat: add K7; Dry throat: add KI6.

2. Depletion of Qi and Blood

1) Principal symptoms and signs

Sallow complexion, shortness of breath, spontaneous perspiration, feebleness, weariness, severe palpitation, insomnia; pale tongue with white and thin coating; thready and relaxed pulse.

These are commonly encountered in patients infected by HIV, or in patients suffering from ARC.

2) Pathogenesis

Shortness of breath, feebleness, weariness, etc. are manifestations of Qi depletion; spontaneous perspiration is due to the failure of consolidative and conservative function of Defence Qi; palpitation and insomnia are caused by the depletion of

Blood, which leads to the malnutrition of Heart.

3) Therapeutic principle

Benefit Qi, nourish Blood.

4) Therapy

Chinese medicinal herbs

① Referential prescription

Decoction for Invigorating Spleen and Nourishing Heart; Decoction Consisting of Eight Precious Ingredients.

② Chinese medicinal herbs commonly used

Radix Astragali seu Hedysari, Radix Codonopsis Pilosulae, Rnizoma Atractylodis Macrocephalac, Rhizoma Rehmanniae Praeparata, Radix Paeoniae Alba, Radix Angelicae Sinensis, Fructus Ziziphi Jujubae, Radix Glycyrrhizae Praeparata.

Formulated preparation: Pill for Invigorating Spleen and Nourishing Heart, 9g, po, tid.

Pill of Eight Precious Ingredients, 9g, po, tid. Bolus of Ten Powerful Tonics, 9g, po, tid. Radix Ginseng Pill for Nourishing Nutrient System, 9g, po, tid.

③ Modification of herbs

Shortness of breath aggravated during physical activities: add Gekko gecko.

Evident palpitation or severe palpitation: add Dens Draconis, Fructus Schisandrae.

Comparatively serious insomnia: add Semen Ziziphi Spinosae, Caulis Polygoni Multiflori.

Profuse night sweat: add Concha Ostreae (charred), Fructus Tritici Levis, Radix Ephedrae.

Acupuncture and moxibustion

① Meridians and acupoints commonly selected

CV4, GV20, ST36; adjunct acupoints: SP6, BL20, BL15; invigorating manipulation.

② Modification of acupoints

Shortness of breath: needle CV6 and cauterize it with moxa.

Palpitation and insomnia: add PC6, HT7.

Diarrhea or defecation of loose stool: cauterize CV8 with moxa.

3. Asthenia and Weakness of Spleen-Stomach

1) Principal symptoms and signs

Listlessness, feebleness, weariness, emaciation, anorexia, poor appetite, feeling of fullness and distension in the epigastrium or abdomen, loose stool or diarrhea; white and thin, or white and greasy coating of the tongue; thready and relaxed pulse.

These are commonly encountered in patients suffering from AIDS or ARC.

2) Pathogenesis

Stomach is in charge of the reception of food; Spleen is responsible for digestion and transportation. Therefore, Asthenia and Weakness of Spleen and Stomach lead to anorexia, feeling of fullness and distension in the abdomen, loose stool, or even diarrhea. Due to the malnutrition and deficiency of Qi and Blood, there are listlessness, feebleness, weariness, and emaciation.

3) Therapeutic principle

Strengthen Spleen, nourish Stomach.

4) Therapy

Chinese medicinal herbs

① Referential prescription

Decoction for Invigorating Middle Energizer and Benefiting Qi.

② Chinese medicinal herbs commonly used

Radix Astragali seu Hedysari, Radix Codonopsis Pilosulae, Rhizoma Atractylodis Macrocephalae, Poria coccos, Rhizoma

Dioscoreae, Radix Bupleuri, Rhizoma Cimicifugae, Semen Dolichoris Album, Semen Coicis.

Formulated preparation: Pill for Invigorating Middle Energizer and Benefiting Qi, 9g, po, bid; Pill for Arousing Spleen, 3g, po, bid or tid.

③ Modification of herbs

Abdominal distension: add Fructus Aurantii, Fructus Amomi, Radix Aucklandiae.

Loose stool or diarrhea: add Fructus Chebulae, Semen Myristicae (roasted).

White, thick, and greasy coating of the tongue: add Rhizoma Atractylodis, Cortex Magnoliae Officinalis.

Acupuncture and moxibustion

① Meridians and acupoints commonly selected

CV12, ST25, ST36; invigorating manipulation.

② Modification of acupoints

Obvious feebleness: add CV4 (moxibustion).

Distension of the abdomen and hypochondriac pain: BL18, LR2.

Comparatively serious abdominal distension and diarrhea: ST37.

4. Asthenia of Liver-Kidney Yin

1) Principal symptoms and signs

Headache, dizziness, tinnitus, dryness of eyes, photophobia, irritability, irascibility, hectic fever, night sweat, aching of the waist, weakness of both legs, loss of hair; reddened tongue with little saliva; thready and bow-string pulse.

These are commonly encountered in patients suffering from AIDS and ARC.

2) Pathogenesis

Headache, irritability, and irascibility are caused by deficiency of Liver-Kidney Yin and upward harassment of asthenic

Fire; insufficient moistening and nourishment result in tinnitus, dryness of eyes; aching of the waist and weakness of legs are due to Kidney Asthenia; hectic fever and night sweat are manifestations of Yin Asthenia.

3) Therapeutic principle

Nourish and tonify Liver-Kidney.

4) Therapy

Chinese medicinal herbs

① Referential prescription

Bolus of Six Drugs Containing Rhizoma Rehmanniae Praeparatae combined with Two Solstices Pill.

② Chinese medicinal herbs commonly used

Radix Rehmanniae, Fructus Corni, Poria coccos, Cortex Moutan Radicis, Radix Paeoniae Alba, Fructus Ligustri Lucidi, Herba Ecliptae, Fructus Lycii.

Formulated preparation: Bolus of Six Drugs containing Rhizoma Rehmanniae Praeparatae combined with Two Solstices Pill, 6-9g, po, bid. Bolus Converging to the Left (Kidney), 9g, po, bid or tid.

③ Modification of herbs

Comparatively serious headache and dizziness (or vertigo): add Concha Haliotidis, Flos Chrysanthemi (Alba), Ramulus Uncariae cum Uncis.

Tinnitus: add Magnetitum.

Dryness of eyes, photophobia, and blurring of vision: add Semen Cassiae, Flos Eriocauli, Fructus Tribuli (Alba).

Irritability and irascibility: add Radix Gentianae, Radix Scutellariae.

Hectic fever and night sweat: add Rhizoma Anemarrhenae, Cortex Phellodendri, Plastrum Testudinis; or add Bolus for Replenishing Yin Greatly, 9g, po, bid, simultaneously.

Nocturnal emission: add Os Draconis, Concha Ostreae,

Fructus Rosae Laevigatae, Stamen Nelumbinis; or add Golden Lock Pill for Consolidating Kidney Essence, 3-6g, po, tid. simultaneously.

Acupuncture and moxibustion

① Meridians and acupoints commonly selected

Principal acupoints: KI3, BL23, SP6. Adjunct acupoints: LR3, GB34.

② Modification of acupoints

Nocturnal emission: add BL52, LR4.

Insomnia: add HT7, PC6.

Dizziness: add GV23.

Night sweat: add KI7.

5. Asthenia of Lung-Kidney Yin

1) Principal symptoms and signs

Dry cough with little phlegm, dryness of the mouth and throat; hectic fever, night sweat, flushing, tinnitus, deafness, aching of the waist, weakness of both legs, nocturnal emission; reddened tongue with little saliva; thready and rapid pulse.

These are commonly encountered in patients suffering from AIDS or ARC.

2) Pathogenesis

There is a mutual promotive relation between Lung and Kidney under normal circumstances. Deficiency of Yin leads to hyperactivity of Yang. Dry cough and dryness of the mouth and throat are caused by Asthenia of Lung Yin; tinnitus, deafness, aching of the waist, and weakness of both legs result from Asthenia of Kidney Yin; hyperactivity of Ministerial Fire elicits nocturnal emission.

3) Therapeutic principle

Nourish and tonify Lung-Kidney.

4) Therapy

Chinese medicinal herbs

① Referential prescription

Decoction of Radix Adenophorae Strictae and Radix Ophiopogonis combined with Bolus for Replenishing Yin Greatly.

② Chinese medicinal herbs commonly used

Radix Glehniae, Radix Ophiopogonis, Rhizoma Polygonati Odorati, Radix Trichosanthis, Radix Rehmanniae, Rhizoma Anemarrhenae, Plastrum Testudinis, Fructus Lycii, Fructus Ligustri Lucidi.

Formulated preparation: Bolus for Eight-Immortals' Longevity, 9g, po, tid. Sweet Dew Bolus for Nourishing Yin, 9g, po, bid.

③ Modification of herbs

Dry cough with little phlegm: add Radix Asteris, Fructus Schisandrae.

Hectic fever and night sweat: add Radix Stellariae, Cortex Lycii Radicis, Rhizoma Picrorhizae.

Tinnitus and deafness: add Rhizoma Rehmanniae Praeparata, Magnetitum.

Acupuncture and moxibustion

① Meridians and acupoints commonly selected

BL13, LU1, KI6, BL23, KI3.

② Modification of acupoints

Tinnitus and deafness: add TE17, ST7.

Aching of the waist and weakness of both legs: add GV4, ST36 (cauterized with moxa).

Night emission: add BL52; invigorating manipulation.

II) Sthenia Syndrome

1. Depression and Stagnation of Liver Qi

1) Principal symptoms and signs

Mental depression, disinclination to speak, feeling of oppression in the chest, distending pain in the hypochondrium, gastric distension, eructation, loss of appetite, irregular defecation, feebleness, weariness; white and thin or white and greasy coating of the tongue; bow-string pulse.

These may be encountered at various stages of AIDS.

2) Pathogenesis

"Liver is fond of reconciliation and extension"; "Liver bears the function of dispersing Qi". When Liver Qi is depressed and stagnated, there will be disorder of Qi mechanism and manifestions of distending pain in the hypochondrium, and eructation, etc.

3) Therapeutic principle

Dredge depressed Liver, disperse stagnated Qi.

4) Therapy

Chinese medicinal herbs

① Referential prescription

Radix Bupleuri Powder for Dispersing Liver Qi

② Chinese medicinal herbs commonly used

Radix Bupleuri, Radix Paeoniae Alba, Fructus Aurantii, Rhizoma Cyperi, Rhizoma Ligustici Chuanxiong, Pericarpium Citri Reticulatae Viride.

Formulated preparation: Pill or Powder for Ease and Free, 9g, po, bid.

③ Modification of herbs

Mental depression: add Rhizoma Acori Graminei, Fructus Citri Sarcodatylis.

Distending pain in the hypochondrium: add Radix Curcumae, Rhizoma Corydalis.

Feeling of epigastric distension and eructation: add Flos Inulae, Caulis Perillae, Calyx Kaki.

Acupuncture and moxibustion

① Meridians and acupoints commonly selected

CV17, LR14, HT7, LR3; reducing manipulation.

② Modification of acupoints

When depressed Qi transforms into Fire: add LI11, LI4.

When melancholy impairs the mind: add PC6.

Asthenia of both Heart and Spleen: add ST36.

2. Internal Accumulation of Wetness-Turbidity

1) Principal symptoms and signs

Lingering high fever, perspiration with sticky sweat, headache as if the head is wrapped, feeling of oppression in the chest, anorexia, aphthosis, erosion of the tongue, unsmooth defecation with sticky, foul, and filthy stool and burning sensation at the anus; yellow and greasy coating of the tongue, or the coating looks like accumulated powder; rapid, weak-floating pulse.

These are commonly encountered in AIDS complicated by casual infections.

2) Pathogenesis

Pestilent Evil cements with Turbidity and accumulates in Middle Energizer. Anorexia and feeling of oppression in the chest is due to the blockage of Qi mechanism. Wetness-Turbidity transforms into Heat, hence there are aphthae and erosion of the tongue. Lucid Apertures are covered by Wetness-Heat-Turbidity, resulting in headache. Foul, sticky stool and burning sensation at the anus are due to the downward flow of Wetness-Heat.

3) Therapeutic principle

Eliminate Turbidity with drugs of fragrant flavour, clear away Heat, resolve Toxin.

4) Therapy

Chinese medicinal herbs

① Referential prescription

Sweet Dew Pellet (Powder) for Detoxification, 6-9 g, po, bid.

② Chinese medicinal herbs commonly used

Herba Agastachis, Herba Artemisiae Scopariae, Rhizoma Acori Graminei, Rhizoma Coptidis, Semen Amomi Cardamomi, Talcum, Rhizoma Belamcandae, Folium Isatidis, Cortex Phellodendri, Radix Paeoniae Rubra.

Formulated preparation: Sweet Dew Pellet for Detoxification, 6-9 g, po, bid.

③ Modification of herbs

Protracted high fever: add Gypsum Fibrosum, Radix Bupleuri.

Distending pain of the head: add Radix Angelicae Dahuricae, Rhizoma Liguistici.

Feeling of oppression in the chest, nausea, vomit: add Rhizoma Pinelliae, Caulis Bambusae in Taeniam.

Sticky stool and burning sensation at the anus: add Radix Puerariae, Rhizoma Coptidis, Cortex Phellodendri.

Aphthae and erosion of the tongue: add Powder of Tin-like Ingredients or Powder of Margarita and Calculus Bovis (local application).

Acupuncture and moxibustion

① Meridians and acupoints commonly selected

LU6, LI4, GV14, TE6; reducing manipulation.

② Modification of acupoints

Comparatively serious Wetness: add SP9.

Nausea and vomit: add CV12.

Sticky stool with burning sensation at the anus: add ST25, LI11.

3. Blazing of Heat-Toxin

1) Principal symptoms and signs

High fever aggravated at night, alleviated by day; profuse perspiration, vexation, restlessness; reddened tongue; thready and rapid pulse. When high fever stirs Blood, there may be multiple blood spots or purplish brown ecchymoses on skin surface or on mucous membrane. When high fever stirs Wind, there may be unconsciousness, delirium, clonic convulsion or twitching.

These are commonly encountered in AIDS patients suffering from casual infection or Kaposi's sarcoma.

2) Pathogenesis

Detained Heat-Toxin consumes Yin; depleted Yin cannot keep Yang. Exuberance of Yang leads to high fever, profuse perspiration, and restlessness. Vexation, unconsciousness, and delirium are due to the attack of Heat-Toxin on Pericardium. Clonic convulsion or twitching is a sign of Wind elicited by high fever. Multiple blood spots are caused by the attack of Heat-Toxin on Blood.

3) Therapeutic principle

Clear away Heat, cool Blood, resolve Toxin.

4) Therapy

Chinese medicinal herbs

① Referential prescription

Decoction for Clearing away Pestilent Evils and Detoxification; Decoction for Clearing away Heat in Nutrient System; Decoction of Cornu Rhinoceri and Radix Rehmanniae.

② Chinese medicinal herbs commonly used

Radix Rehmanniae, Radix Paeoniae Rubra, Cortex Moutan Radicis, Fructus Forsythiae, Flos Lonicerae, Radix Scutellariae, Cornu Rhinoceri, Radix Scrophulariae, Folium Isatidis, Radix Isatidis.

Formulated preparation: Pellet of Miraculous Rhinoceros Horn, 9g, po, qd or bid.

③ Modification of herbs

High fever: add Gypsum Fibrosum, Rhizoma Anemarrhenae.

Blood spots: add Herba seu Radix Cirsii Japonici, Herba Cephalanoploris, Herba Ecliptae, Rhizoma Imperatae, Nodus Nelumbinis Rhizomatis, Radix Sanguisorbae, or Flos Sophorae according to different locale of hemorrhage.

Vexation and restlessness: add Rhizoma Coptidis, Plumula Nelumbinis.

Unconsciousness: add Rhizoma Acori Graminei, Radix Curcumae.

Convulsion or twitching: add Ramulus Uncariae cum Uncis, Scorpio, Scolopendra.

Formulated preparation: Bezoar Bolus (or Powder) for Resurrection, 1.6g, po, bid or tid; Purplish Snow (Powder or Pellet), 1.5-3.0g, po, bid.

Acupuncture and moxibustion

① Meridians and acupoints commonly selected

GV14, LI11, LI4, PC6; reducing manipulation.

② Modification of acupoints

Delirium or convulsion: add GV26, Ex-UE11 (Shixuan); bleed Ex-UE11.

4. Lucid Aperture Covered by Phlegm

1) Principal symptoms and signs

Trance, amnesia, dementia, epilepsy at times; vertigo, dizziness, aching of the waist, weakness of legs; reddened tongue with greasy coating; thready and bow-string or soft, floating, and rapid pulse.

These are commonly encountered in AIDS patients complicated by Cryptococcus, Toxoplasma infection, or in those whose brain tissues are invaded by HIV directly.

2) Pathogenesis

Trance, amnesia, and dementia are due to the covering of Lucid Aperture by Phlegm, which is produced through the scorching effect of Pestilent Heat on body fluids. Vertigo and dizziness are caused by the upward harassment of asthenic Yang, resulting from the deficiency of Liver-Kidney Yin. Aching of the waist and weakness of legs are manifestations of Kidney Asthenia or Marrow Sea deficiency.

3) Therapeutic principle

Clear away Heat, resolve Phlegm, nourish Yin, promote resuscitation.

4) Therapy

Chinese medicinal herbs

① Referential prescription

Decoction for Replenishing Primordial Essence Greatly combined with Decoction for Eliminating Phlegm.

② Chinese medicinal herbs commonly used

Radix Rehmanniae, Rhizoma Dioscoreae, Fructus Corni, Fructus Lycii, Concha Ostreae, Carapax Trionycis, Rhizoma Pinelliae, Arisaema cum Bile, Rhizoma Acori Graminei, Fructus Aurantii Immaturus.

Formulated preparations may also be selected, such as Pill for Clearing Away Heart Fire and Expelling Phlegm, 3g, po, bid.

③ Modification of herbs

Trance: add Succinum, Radix Polygalae, Poria cum Ligno Hospite.

Vertigo or dizziness: add Rhizoma Gastrodiae, Ramulus Uncariae cum Uncis, Scorpio.

Dementia and amnesis: add Radix Curcumae, Concretio Silicea Bambusae;

Aching of the waist and weakness of legs: add Placenta Hominis Bolus for Energetic Rehabilitation, 9g, po, bid.

Acupuncture and moxibustion

Needle CV12, HT7, SP6, KI3; or BL15, BL18, BL20, ST40; or alternately.

5. Phlegm Agglutination and Blood Stasis

1) Principal symptoms and signs

Palpable mass or lump under the hypochondrium (hepatosplenomegaly), obstinate nodules (lymphadenectasis), neoplasm, sallow or dimly blackish complexion, listlessness, feebleness; dimly purplish tongue with or without ecchymoses; thready and uneven pulse.

These are commonly encountered in AIDS patients accompanied with Kaposi's sarcoma or other neoplasms.

2) Pathogenesis

Detained Pestilent Toxin impairs Healthy Energy. Phlegm agglutination results from the failure of Spleen transportation and transformation; Asthenia of Qi leads to Blood stasis. The above-mentioned symptoms and signs are manifestations of Phlegm agglutination combined with Blood stasis.

3) Therapeutic principle

Activate Blood, eliminate Phlegm, remove Toxin, resolve stagnation.

4) Therapy

Chinese medicinal herbs

① Referential prescription

Decoction of Four Drugs with Semen Persicae and Flos Carthami combined with Pill for Resolving Scrofula.

② Chinese medicinal herbs commonly used

Rhizoma Rehmanniae Praeparatae, Rhizoma Ligustici Chuanxiong, Radix Paeoniae Rubra, Semen Persicae, Flos Carthami, Rhizoma Zedoariae, Rhizoma Arisaematis, Rhizoma Pinelliae, Bulbus Cremastrae, Concha Ostreae, Bulbus Fritillariae.

③ Modification of herbs

Hepatosplenomegaly: add Rhizoma Sparganii, Carapax Trionycis; or Pill of Decocted Carapax Trionycis, 6-9g, po, bid.

Lymphadenectasis: add Radix Semiaquilegiae, Squama Manitis (fried with liquid adjuvants); or Minor "Golden" Pellet, 0.6g, po, bid.

Neoplasms: Herba Oldenlandiae Diffusae, Herba Scutellariae Barbatae, Rhizoma Zedoariae, Paris polyphylla, Solanum Lyratum Thunb, Herba Agrimoniae, Herba Solani Nigri, Radix Actinidiae Chinensis, Rhizoma Smilacis Glabrae, etc. The following formulated preparations may also be selected: Bolus of Western Calculus Bovis, 3 g, po, bid; Pill of Six Miraculous Drugs, 10 grains, po, bid; Pill of Venenum Bufonis, 5-15 grains, po, bid.

Acupuncture and moxibustion

Needle BL17, BL20, BL23, SP6, LR13, GB25, ST40, LI4; Cauterize ST36, BL43, CV4 with moxa.

II. Treatment of AIDS according to Its Prominent Symptoms and Signs as well as Its Complications

In view of the fact that many foreign doctors have not got mastery of TCM and the disease condition of AIDS is extremely variable and complicated, we write this part of the book and hope it may be of some help to medical workers outside China in treating AIDS.

I) Fever

Fever is often seen in patients suffering from AIDS or ARC. It may be intermittent or persistent, usually caused by casual infection or by unknown reasons. It is aggravated in the afternoon or at night and reaches 38-40°C, accompanied with spontaneous perspiration or night sweat. If it is caused by casual infection, there will be manifestations of the impairment of relevant Viscera. According to TCM, fever may be asthenic or sthenic;

their clinical symptoms and signs and their therapeutic measures are different.

1. Fever due to Yin Asthenia

1) Principal manifestations

Afternoon or nocturnal fever, vexation, hotness at palms and soles, restlessness, night sweat, insomnia, dreaminess, palpitation, dryness of the mouth and throat, mental weariness, feebleness; reddened tongue with little saliva; thready and rapid pulse.

2) Pathogenesis

Tidal fever, night sweat, and reddened tongue signify Internal Heat caused by Yin deficiency; vexation, palpitation, insomnia, dreaminess, etc., are due to the harassment of Heart by asthenic Heat; dryness of the mouth and throat, scanty of saliva results from dificiency of body fluids.

3) Therapeutic principle

Nourish Yin, clear away Heat.

4) Therapy

Chinese medicinal herbs

① Referential prescription

Powder for Clearing Away Hectic Fever combined with Decoction of Radix Angelicae Sinensis for Replenishing Blood.

② Chinese medicinal herbs commonly used

Radix Stellariae, Rhizoma Anemarrhenae, Radix Gentianae Macrophyllae, Herba Artemisiae Chinghao, Cortex Lycii Radicis, Carapax Trionycis, Radix Astragali seu Hedysari, Radix Angelicae Sinensis.

③ Modification of herbs

Vexation and insomnia: add Semen Ziziphi Spinosae, Semen Biotae, Caulis Polygoni Multiflori.

Obvious night sweat: add Concha Ostreae, Fructus Tritici Levis, Radix Oryzae Glutionsae.

Ordinary or severe palpitation: add Poria cum Ligro Hospite, Radix Polygalae, Fructus Schisandrae.

Dizziness: add Radix Angelicae Sinensis, Radix Paeoniae Alba, Flos Chrysanthemi (Alba), Fructus Lycii.

Dryness of the mouth and throat: add Radix Scrophulariae, Radix Adenophorae Strictae, Radix Asparagi, Radix Ophiopogonis.

Dry cough with little phlegm: add Radix Adenophorae Strictae, Radix Ophiopogonis, Bulbus Lilii.

Alopecia: add Fructus Ligustri Lucidi, Radix Polygoni Multiflori Praeparata, Herba Ecliptae.

Acupuncture and moxibustion

① Meridians and acupoints commonly selected

GV14, LI11, LI4, KI3, SP6; uniform invigorating-reducing manipulation.

② Modification of acupoints

Night sweat: add SI3, HT6.

Insomnia and dreaminess: add HT7, LR3, BL15.

Dizziness: add BL18, BL23, GV20, SP6.

Dry cough with little phlegm: add LU5, BL13.

2. Fever due to Asthenia of Qi

1) Principal symptoms and signs

High or low fever aggravated after overwork, feebleness, weariness, shortness of breath, disinclination to speak, poor appetite, loose stool, spontaneous perspiration, liability to catch cold; pale tongue with white and thin coating; weak pulse.

2) Pathogenesis

Shortness of breath, disinclination to speak, feebleness, weariness, etc. are due to the deficiency of Qi, fever is caused by the outward floating of asthenic Yang; spontaneous perspiration and liability to catch cold result from the weakness of Defence Qi.

3) Therapeutic principle

Invigorate Middle Energizer, benefit Qi, clear away fever with drugs of sweet flavour and warm nature.

4) Therapy

Chinese medicinal herbs

① Referential prescription

Decoction for Invigorating Middle Energizer and Benefiting Qi.

② Chinese medicinal herbs commonly used

Radix Codonopsis Pilosulae, Radix Astragali seu Hedysari, Radix Angelicae Sinensis, Rhizoma Atractylodis Macrocephalae, Rhizoma Cimicifugae, Radix Bupleuri, Radix Glycyrrhizae.

Formulated preparation: Bolus for Invigorating Middle Energizer and Benefiting Qi, 6-9g, po, bid or tid.

③ Modification of herbs

Spontaneous perspiration: add Fructus Tritici Levis, Concha Ostreae, Radix Oryzae Glutinosae.

Aversion to wind during perspiration: add Ramulus Cinnamomi, Radix Paeoniae Alba.

Feeling of fullness and oppression in the chest and epigastrium, accompanied with white and greasy coating of the tongue: add Rhizoma Atractylodis, Poria coccos, Cortex Magnoliae Officinalis.

Loose stool and cold limbs: add Rhizoma Zingiberis (baked), Cortex Cinnamomi.

Acupuncture and moxibustion

① Meridians and acupoints commonly selected

GV14, LI11, LI4, BL20, ST36; uniform invigorating-reducing manipulation.

② Modification of acupoints

Spontaneous perspiration: add KI7.

Poor appetite, loose stool: add SP4, ST25; cauterize CV8 with moxa.

Shortness of breath, feebleness: cauterize CV4 and CV6 with moxa.

3. Fever due to infection

1) Principal symptoms and signs

High fever, thirst, profuse perspiration, cough with sticky phlegm, even accompanied by hidden macule and papule, epistaxis, hematochezia, unconsciousness, clonic convulsion or twitching; yellow coating of the tongue or reddened tongue with little coating; full and rapid pulse.

2) Pathogenesis

Deficiency of Healthy Energy, invasion of Pestilent Toxin; their wrestling results in fever and perspiration. Exuberance and blockage of Lung Heat lead to cough with sticky phlegm. Bleeding disorders are caused by Blood Heat. Unconsciousness signifies Pericardium is attacked by Evil Heat; twitching signifies the stirring of Wind by Heat.

3) Therapeutic principle

Clear away Heat, cool Blood, resolve Toxin.

4) Therapy

Chinese medicinal herbs

① Referential prespiration

Powder of Fructus Forsythiae and Flos Lonicerae; White Tiger Decoction; Decoction for Clearing Away Heat in Nutrient System.

② Chinese medicinal herbs commonly used

Flos Lonicerae, Herba Taraxaci, Herba Violae, Gypsum Fibrosum, Cornu Rhinoceri, Radix Scrophulariae, Radix Isatidis, Folium Isatidis, Herba Houttuyniae.

③ Modification of herbs

Cough with yellow or purulent phlegm: add Rhizoma Phragmitis, Semen Armeniacae Amarum, Semen Benincasae, Radix Scutellariae.

Constipation with yellow and dry coating of the tongue: add Radix et Rhizoma Rhei, Natrii Sulfas.

Hidden skin eruption: add Radix Paeoniae Rubra, Cortex Moutan Radicis, Radix Arnebiae seu Lithospermi, Radix Rubiae.

Epistaxis: add Rhizoma Imperatae, Nodus Nelumbinis Rhizomatis.

Hematuria: add Herba Cephalanoploris.

Hematochezia (Hemafecia): add Flos Sophorae, Radix Sanguisorbae.

High fever, unconsciousness, twitching: select Bezoar Bolus for Resurrection, 1 bolus, po, qd or bid; or Pellet of Precious Drugs, 3-5 pellets, po, bid or tid.

Acupuncture and moxibustion

① Meridians and acupoints commonly selected

GV14, LI11, LI4, TE1; strong stimulation and reducing manipulation; bleed LU11, LI1.

② Modification of acupoints

Cough caused by Lung Heat: add BL12, LU7.

Nutrient-Blood System invaded by Heat: add HT9, PC9, PC7, SP6.

Unconsciousness: add GV26, KI1, Ex-UE11 (Shixuan).

II) Diarrhea

During prodromal stage of AIDS or in patients whose illness develops into AIDS swiftly, 50-90% of them are accompanied with diarrhea and their body weight loses progressively. Such diarrhea may be intermittent or persistent. It may be caused by specific bacteria, protozoa, or other pathogens in some patients; while in other patients, the cause is unknown. Diarrhea in AIDS may be divided into two types: the Spleen Asthenia and the Wetness-Heat.

1. Diarrhea caused by Spleen Asthenia

1) Principal symptoms and signs

Sometimes diarrhea, sometimes loose stool; poor appetite, feeling of fullness and distension in the epigastrium or abdomen; sallow complexion, emaciation, weariness, feebleness; pale tongue with white coating; thready and weak pulse.

2) Pathogenesis

Stomach is in charge of the reception of food; Spleen is in charge of the transportation and transformation of nutrients. Thus, poor appetite and feeling of fullness and distension of the epigastrium are caused by Stomach Asthenia; loose stool and abdominal distension are caused by Spleen Asthenia, Emaciation and feebleness result from the deficiency of Qi and Blood.

3) Therapeutic principle

Strengthen Spleen, eliminate Wetness.

4) Therapy

Chinese medicinal herbs

① Referential prescription

Powder of Radix Ginseng, Poria coccos, and Rhizoma Atractylodis Macrocephalae.

② Chinese medicinal herbs commonly used

Radix Ginseng (Radix Codonopsis Pilosulae), Rhizoma Atractylodis Macrocephalae. Poria coccos, Rhizoma Dioscoreae, Semen Coicis, Semen Dolichoris Album, Semen Nelumbinis, Pericarpium Citri Reticulatae.

Formulated preparation: Powder of Radix Ginseng, Poria coccos, and Rhizoma Atractylodis Macrocephalae, 9 g, po, bid.

③ Modification of herbs

Fullness and distension of the epigastrium: add Fructus Aurantii, Fructus Crataegi, Massa Fermentata Medicinalis,

Semen Raphani.

Abdominal distension: add Pericarpium Arecae, Radix Saussureae Lappae.

Abdominal pain: add Radix Paeoniae Alba (parched), Radix Glycyrrhizae (fried with liquid adjuvants), Rhizoma Corydalis.

Abdominal pain and diarrhea before dawn: add Fructus Psoraleae, Semen Myristicae, Rhizoma Zingiberis (roasted); or Pill of Four Miraculous Drugs, 9 g, po, qd or bid.

Acupuncture and moxibustion

① Meridians and acupoints commonly selected

BL20, LR13, ST25; CV8, ST36 (cauterize with moxa).

② Modification of acupoints

Poor appetite and epigastric distension: add CV12;

Kidney Asthenia: cauterize GV4 and CV4 with moxa.

2. Diarrhea caused by Wetness-Heat

1) Principal symptoms and signs

Abdominal pain, urgent diarrhea, tenesmus or unsmooth defecation; foul and yellowish brown stool, or mixed with pus and blood; burning hot sensation at the anus; dysphoria with feverish sensation, thirst; oliguria; yellow and greasy coating of the tongue; slippery and rapid or weak-floating and rapid pulse.

2) Pathogenesis

Wetness is heavy and turbid in nature; when Wetness is glued to Heat, and they stick together, blocking Qi Mechanism, the intestinal tract is compelled to discharge. Therefore, there are abdominal pain, tenesmus, urgent diarrhea. Wetness-Heat is sticky, leading to unsmooth defecation. Dysphoria with feverish sensation, thirst, and burning sensation at the anus are caused by Wetness-Heat.

3) Therapeutic principle

Clear away Heat, eliminate Wetness.

4) Therapy

Chinese medicinal herbs

① Referential prescription

Decoction of Radix Puerariae, Radix Scutellariae, and Rhizoma Coptidis; Radix Pulsatillae Decoction.

② Chinese medicinal herbs commonly used

Radix Puerariae, Radix Scutellariae, Rhizoma Coptidis, Radix Pulsatillae, Herba Patriniae, Cortex Fraxini, Radix Sophorae Flavescentis.

③ Modification of herbs

Feeling of epigastric or abdominal oppression and distension, accompanied with yellow, thick, and greasy coating of the tongue: add Rhizoma Atractylodis, Cortex Magnoliae Officinalis.

Abdominal pain, sticky stool, unsmooth defecation: add Radix et Rhizoma Rhei, Semen Arecae, Radix Aucklandiae.

Stool mixed with obvious pus and blood: add Radix Sanguisorbae, Radix Paeoniae Rubra, Herba Taraxaci.

Acupuncture and moxibustion

ST25, ST36, ST44, SP9; reducing manipulation.

III) Skin lesion

Itching and skin eruptions are often encountered in patients suffering from AIDS or ARC. Manifestations of skin eruptions may be nonspecific maculopapule, eczema, herpes simplex, or herpes zoster.

1. Cutaneous pruritus

1) Principal symptoms and signs

Dryness and itching of the skin with white furfures, or reddened skin with blood spots after scratching; fever, dry mouth, vexation, constipation, deep-coloured urine, pale complexion, feebleness, weariness; reddened tongue or pale red tongue with white or yellow thin coating; thready and rapid pulse.

2) Pathogenesis

Depletion of Yin and Blood transforms into Dryness and Wind, resulting in dryness and itching of the skin. Fever, vexation, and deep-coloured urine are caused by Interior Heat, which is the consequence of Yin-Blood deficiency. Pale complexion, feebleness, and weariness are due to Qi Asthenia and Blood Asthenia, since Qi and Blood come from the same origin.

3) Therapeutic principle

Nourish Blood, moisten Dryness, cool Blood, clear away Heat.

4) Therapy

Chinese medicinal herbs

① Referential prescription

Prescription for Nourishing Blood to Stop Wind; Prescription for Relieving Itching and Calming Wind.

② Chinese medicinal herbs commonly used

Radix Astragali seu Hedysari, Radix Angelicae Sinensis, Radix Paeoniae Alba, Radix Paeoniae Rubra, Rhizoma Ligustici Chuanxiong, Radix Rehmanniae, Cortex Moutan Radicis, Radix Scrophulariae, Flos Carthami, Fructus Tribuli (Alba).

③ Modification of herbs

Comparatively serious Blood Heat: add Radix Polygoni Multiflori, Radix Asparagi, Radix Ophiopogonis, Fructus Ligustri Lucidi.

Comparatively serious Blood Asthenia: add Rhizoma Rehmanniae Praeparatae, Radix Angelicae Sinensis, Colla Corii Asini.

Concurrent Blood stasis: add Radix Salviae Miltiorrhizae, Semen Persicae.

Acupuncture and moxibustion

① Meridians and acupoints commonly selected

SP10, ST36, BL17, invigorating manipulation.

LI11, LI4, SP6; reducing manipulation.

② Modification of acupoints

Itching of the scalp: add GB20.

Itching of the vulva or scrotum: add LR3 or LR5.

Itching of the anus: add GV1, BL57.

2. Eczema

1) Principal symptoms and signs

Cutaneous erythema, papule, blister; paroxysmal itching; oozing or erosion, ulceration after being scratched; anorexia, feeling of oppression in the chest; or fever, yellow and greasy coating of the tongue; weak-floating and rapid pulse.

2) Pathogenesis

The skin and superficial venules are invaded by Wetness-Heat Evil, resulting in oozing, erosion, or ulceration. Anorexia and feeling of oppression in the chest are caused by internal accumulation of Wetness-Heat.

3) Therapeutic principle

Clear away Heat, eliminate Wetness.

4) Therapy

Chinese medicinal herbs

① Referential prescription

Wen's Experiential Prescription.

② Chinese medicinal herbs commonly used

Radix Gentianae, Rhizoma Atractylodis, Cortex Phellodendri, Cortex Dictamni Radicis, Rhizoma Smilacis Glabrae, Fructus Kochiae, Flos Lonicerae, Bombyx Batryticatus, Periostracum Cicadae, Excrementum Bombycis, corium Erinacei.

③ Modification of herbs

Serious dominance of Wetness: add Rhizoma Dioscoreae Hypoglaucae, Rhizoma Alismatis, Semen Coicis.

Serious dominance of fever: add Radix Scutellariae, Fructus Gardeniae.

Acupuncture and moxibustion

Principal acupoints: LI11, SP10, SP6. Adjunct acupoints: GV14, TE6, LR14, LI4, GB31; reducing manipulation.

3. Herpes zoster

1) Principal symptoms and signs

Appearance of clusters of blisters on the abdomen, back, chest, or face, accompanied with serious pain, even hemorrhagic spots or bloody vesicles; bitter taste, dysphoria, feeling of oppression in the epigastrium, anorexia; yellow and greasy coating of the tongue; bow-string and rapid pulse or weak-floating and rapid pulse.

2) Pathogenesis

Internal accumulation of Wetness-Heat results in feeling of oppression in the epigastrium and anorexia; blockage of Nutrient-Defence System by Wetness-Heat in the superficies of the body leads to blisters; bitter taste and dysphoria are caused by the exuberance of Liver-Gallbladder Fire.

3) Therapeutic principle

Clear away Heat, purge Liver, eliminate Wetness, cool Blood.

4) Therapy

Chinese medicinal herbs

① Referential prescription

Decoction of Radix Gentianae for Purging Liver Fire.

② Chinese medicinal herbs commonly used

Radix Bupleuri, Radix Scutellariae, Fructus Gardeniae, Poris coccos, Rhizoma Alismatis, Cortex Moutan Radicis, Radix Paeoniae Rubra, Indigo Naturalis, Folium Isatidis.

③ Modification of herbs

Fever: add Flos Lonicerae, Fructus Forsythiae.

Flushing, bitter taste: add Radix Rehmanniae, Rhizoma Anemarrhenae.

Dysphoria and irascibility: add Rhizoma Coptidis, Herba Lophatheri.

Hemorrhage or accompanied with bloody vesicles: add Radix Scrophulariae, Radix Arnebiae seu Lithospermi.

Anorexia and feeling of oppression in the epigastrium: add Rhizoma Pinelliae, Fructus Amomi.

Acupuncture and moxibustion

① Meridians and acupoints commonly selected

LI11, LI4, SP10, SP6, LR2, LR14; reducing manipulation.

② Modification of acupoints

Herpes on the chest, hypochondria, or lateral abdomen: add GB34.

Herpes on the back: add BL40.

Serious pain: add TE6.

IV) Systemic lymphadenopathy

Systemic lymphadenopathy of unknown cause is closely related to AIDS, it is also a part of clinical manifestation of AIDS.

1. Principal symptoms and signs

Fever, night sweat, feebleness, weariness, aching of muscles; lymphadenectasis with or without tenderness; hepatosplenomegaly in some of these patients; reddened tongue with yellow and thin coating; thready and bow-string pulse.

2. Pathogenesis

Deficiency of Kidney Yin and depletion of Qi and Blood; dificiency of Yin brings about Internal Heat, which scorches body fluids and Wetness, thereby Phlegm occurs and accumulates. According to TCM, Lymphadenectasis and hepatosplenomegaly are manifestations of Phlegm agglutination. Feebleness and weariness are due to the deficiency of Healthy Energy.

3. Threapeutic principle

Nourish Yin, clear away Heat, resolve Phlegm, disperse agglutination.

4. Therapy

1) Chinese medicinal herbs

Referential prescription

Bolus for Resolving Scrofula Interiorly.

Chinese medicinal herbs commonly used

Spica Prunellae, Sargassum tortile, Radix Trichosanthis, Radix Scrophulariae, Radix Rehmanniae, Fructus Forsythiae, Radix Ampelopsis, Bulbus Cremastrae, Concha Meretricis seu Cyclinae, Radix Semiaquilegiae, Radix Asparagi, Radix Ophiopogonis.

Formulated preparation: For scrofula, Bolus for Resolving Scrofula Interiorly, 6-9 g, po, bid; or Minor Golden Pellet, 0.6-1.2 g, po, bid. For Hepatosplenomegaly, Pill of Decocted Carapax Trionycis, 6-9 g, po, bid.

Modification of herbs

Feeling of stuffiness and oppression in the chest and epigastrium due to the stagnation of Liver Qi; add Radix Bupleuri, Pericarpium Citri Reticulatae Viride, Pericarpium Citri Reticulatae.

Shortness of breath, feebleness, glossy pale complexion due to Asthenia of Spleen Qi: add Radix Astragali seu Hedysari, Radix Codonopsis Pilosulae, Poria coccos, Rhizoma Pinelliae.

Dizziness: add Fructus Ligustri Lucidi, Herba Ecliptae, Fructus Lycii.

Obvious lymphadenectasis: add Concha Ostreae (unprocessed), Concha Arcae (calcined), Rhizoma Dioscoreae Bulbiferae, Squama Manitis (fried with liquid adjuvants).

Concurrent Blood Stasis: add Semen Persicae, Radix Salviae Miltiorrhizae.

2) Acupuncture and moxibustion

Meridians and acupoints commonly selcted

BL23, KI3, ST40, SP10, SP6, Ashi (Oh Yes) acupoint; uniform invigorating and reducing manipulation; or cauterize GV14, TE10 with moxa simultaneously.

Modification of acupoints

Feeling of stuffiness and oppression in the chest and epigastrium: add LR14.

Feebleness and poor appetite: add ST36, BL20.

Low fever and night sweat: add LI11, LI4, HT6, KI7.

V) Encephalitis and/or meningitis

The CNS of patients suffering from AIDS is apt to be infected by pathogens casually. Pathogens most commonly encountered are toxoplasma, cryptococcus, etc. According to different manifestations of symptoms and signs, such infections are divided into two types.

1. Asthenia of Liver-Kidney Yin

1) Principal symptoms and signs

Fever, headache, dizziness (vertigo), tinnitus, hypomnesia, visual disturbance, aching of the waist and weakness of legs, numbness of limbs, quivering, walking with unsteady steps; reddened tongue with little coating; thready and uneven pulse.

2) Pathogenesis

Fever results from Yin Asthenia; headache and dizziness are due to the upward harassment of Liver Wind; visual disturbance is caused by the malnutrition of eyes; hypomnesia comes from the malnutrition of Heart; numbness and quivering are due to the malnutrition of Tendons; aching of the waist and weakness of legs are manifestations of the deficiency of Kidney Essence.

3) Therapeutic principle

Nourish and tonify Liver-Kidney, foster Yin, calm Wind.

4) Therapy

Chinese medicinal herbs

① Referential prescription

Bolus for Replenishing Yin Greatly combined with Bolus of Fructus Lycii-Flos Chrysanthemi and Rhizoma Rehmanniae Praeparatae.

② Chinese medicinal herbs commonly used

Plastrum Testudinis, Radix Rehmanniae, Rhizoma Rehmanniae Praeparatae, Radix Polygoni Multiflori, Fructus Corni, Fructus Lucii, Rhizoma Anemarrhenae, Cortex Phellodendri, Flos Chrysanthemi (Alba), Ramulus Uncariae cum Uncis, Concha Ostreae.

Formulated preparation: Bolus for Replenishing Yin Greatly, 9 g, po, bid or tid; Bolus of Fructus Lycii-Flos Chrysanthemi and Rhizoma Rehmanniae Praeparatae , 9 g, po, bid.

③ Modification of herbs

Headache: add Bombyx Batryticatus, Buthus martensi.

Dizziness (vertigo): add Rhizoma Gastrodiae, Fructus Tribuli (Alba).

Blurring of vision: add Fructus Ligustri Lucidi, Flos Eriocauli.

Numbness and/or quivering of limbs: add Radix Paeoniae Alba, Radix Angelicae Sinensis, Radix Achyranthis Bidentatae, Lumbricus.

Weakness of limbs: add Bolus for Walking with Energetic Strides, 9 g, po, bid.

Acupuncture and moxibustion

① Meridians and acupoints commonly selected

GV16, LI11, LI4, ST36, LR3; uniform invigorating and reducing manipulation.

② Modification of acupoints

Headache and dizziness: add KI3, GV20.

Numbness and weakness of limbs: add BL18, BL23, GB39, SP9.

2. Blockage caused by Phlegm stagnation

1) Principal symptoms and signs

Fever, headache or dizziness (vertigo), disturbance of consciousness, dysphasia or hemiplegia, or onset of epilepsy now and then, weariness, feebleness; dim, purplish reddened tongue with little coating or yellow and greasy coating; bow-string and rapid pulse.

2) Pathogenesis

There are Asthenia of Liver-Kidney Yin and deficiency of Qi and Blood. Asthenic fever results from Yin Asthenia. Debility of Qi leads to Blood stasis, while body fluid scorched by Heat brings about Phlegm. The combination of stagnated Blood and Phlegm blocks Collaterals at the root of the tongue, resulting in dysphasia. Hemiplegia is caused by the obstruction of Meridians and Collaterals. Headache and dizziness are due to the upward harassment of Asthenic Wind. Disturbance of consciousness signifies the confusion of Lucid Apertures. Epilepsy is precipitated by the upward raid of Liver Wind intermingled with Phlegm.

3) Therapeutic principle

Nourish Yin, retrieve Yang, activate Blood, eliminate Phlegm.

4) Therapy

Chinese medicinal herbs

① Referential prescription

Pill for Calming Epilepsy; Decoction for Opening Aperture and Activating Blood.

② Chinese medicinal herbs commonly used

Radix Rehmanniae, Rhizoma Gastrodiae, Bulbus Fritillariae Cirrhosae, Arisaema cum Bile, Rhizoma Pinelliae, Rhizoma Acori Graminei, Plastrum Testudinis, Radix Salviae Miltiorrhizae, Semen Persicae, Succinum.

③ Modification of herbs

Dominance of fever: add Radix Gentianae, Rhizoma Coptidis.

Headache, dizziness: add Fructus Tribuli (Alba), Spica Prunellae, Concha Haliotidis.

Dysphasia: add Concretio Silicea Bambusae and Radix Curcumae to Radix Rehmanniae Decoction.

Disturbance of consciousness, epilepsy, accompanied with abundant phlegm: add Pill of Alumen and Radix Curcumae, 1.5 g, po, bid.

Blood Stasis: add Radix Paeoniae Rubra, Lumbricus, Rhizoma Ligustici Chuanxiong.

Hemiplegia: add Bolus for Rehabilitation, 9 g, po, bid.

All AIDS accompanied with CNS infection: add Purplish Golden Lozenge, 0.3-0.6 g po, qd or bid. This formulated preparation may ward off Filth, resolve Toxin, eliminate Phlegm, and promote resuscitation.

Acupuncture and moxibustion

GV20, HT7, LR3, KR3, GI20, SB40, PC6; uniform invigorating and reducing manipulation.

VI) Dyspnea and chest pain

Mostly, these are manifestations of Pneumocystis carinii pneumonia. Expectoration of sputum mixed with pus and blood signifies the existence of bacterial infection. According to TCM, they are divided into two types.

1. Dryness-Heat due to Yin Asthenia

1) Principal symptoms and signs

Fever, perspiration, dry cough or cough with little phlegm. In seirous cases, there are successive cough, dyspnea, chest and hypochondriac pain, or accompanied with hemoptysis; dryness of the nose, mouth, and throat, sore throat; reddened tongue with little coating or yellow and thin coating; thready and rapid pulse.

2) Pathogenesis

Dryness-Heat are generated by the depletion of Essence and Blood. Dry cough, dryness of the nose, mouth, and the throat, fever, perspiration, reddened tongue, and yellow coating of the tongue, all these are manifestations of Dryness-Heat caused by Yin deficiency.

3) Therapeutic principle

Nourish Yin, moisten Dryness, astringe Lung, stop cough.

4) Therapy

Chinese medicinal herbs

① Referential prescription

Decoction of Radix Asparagi, Radix Ophiopogonis, Rhizoma Anemarrhenae, and Bulbus Fritillariae; combined with Bolus for Eight-Immortals Longevity.

② Chinese medicinal herbs commonly used

Radix Rehmanniae, Radix Asparagi, Radix Ophiopogonis, Rhizoma Anemarrhenae, Bulbus Fritillariae, Fructus Corni, Cortex Mori Radicis, Fructus Schisandrae, Radix Asteris, Radix Glehniae.

③ Modification of herbs

Fever: add Fructus Gardeniae, Fructus Forsythiae.

Sore throat: add Radix Scrophulariae, Lasiosphaera seu Calvatia.

Cough, dyspnea: add Fructus Perillae, Gekko gecko.

Chest pain: add Radix Rubiae, Flos Inulae.

Aching of the waist and weakness of legs: add Fructus Lycii,

Radix Achyranthis Bidentatae.

Acupuncture and moxibustion

① Meridians and acupoints commonly selected

LU7, LU5, KI3, CV22, BL23; uniform invigorating and reducing manipulation.

② Modification of acupoints

Dry throat: add KI6.

Hemoptysis: add LU6.

Fever: add LI4, LU10.

2. Phlegm-Heat accumulated in Lung

1) Principal symptoms and signs

Fever, perspiration, cough with yellow and sticky phlegm or sputum mixed with blood; feeling of oppression in the chest or chest pain, even dyspnea; yellow and greasy coating of the tongue, slippery and rapid pulse.

2) Pathogenesis

Phlegm-Heat accumulate in Lung. The purifying and descending function of Lung is impaired. Hence there are cough and yellow sputum. When Lung Collaterals are damaged, there will be hemoptysis. Feeling of oppression in the chest, chest pain, and dyspnea are caused by the blockage of Qi mechanism.

3) Therapeutic principle

Clear away Heat, clean Lung, resolve Phlegm, stop cough.

4) Therapy

Chinese medicinal herbs

① Referential prescription

Pill for Clearing Away Lung Heat and Resolving Phlegm.

② Chinese medicinal herbs commonly used

Radix Scutellariae, Fructus Gardeniae, Flos Lonicerae, Herba Taraxaci, Semen Trichosanthis, Cortex Mori Radicis, Bulbus Fritillariae, Poria coccos, Semen Coicis, Exocarpium

Citri Grandis.

③ Modification of drugs

High fever, yellow sputum: add Herba Houttuyniae, Succus Bambosae, Gypsum Fibrosum; Powder of Indigo Naturalis and Concha Meretricis seu Cyclinae.

Dyspnea with feeling of fullness in the chest: add Semen Lepidii seu Descurainiae.

Chest pain, feeling of oppression in the chest: add Flos Inulae, Radix Rubiae.

Acupuncture and moxibustion

① Meridians and acupoints commonly selected

BL13, LU5, LI11, LI4, ST40; reducing manipulation.

② Modification of acupoints

Fever: add GV14.

Chest pain: add PC6, TE6.

VII) Kaposi's sarcoma

Kaposi's sarcoma usually occurs on human cutaneous superficies or within the oral cavity; it is an important clinical manifestation of AIDS and may be regarded as its diagnostic basis.

1. Principal symptoms and signs

Pale or purplish red nodule(s) or lump(s) on cutaneous superficies, or within the oral cavity, without pain; hectic fever, night sweat, dizziness, aching of the waist, feebleness, emaciation. lymphadenectasis; reddened tongue with little coating; thready and rapid pulse.

2. Pathogenesis

Hyperactivity of Fire due to Yin deficiency; Blood Collaterals and extravasated blood are scorched by Fire; thus malignant nodule(s) or lump(s) appears. Dizziness, aching of the waist, feebleness, and emaciation are caused by the deficiency of Essence and Blood; hectic fever and night sweat result from the deficiency of Yin.

3. Therapeutic principle

Nourish Yin, cool Blood, eliminate Stasis, resolve Toxin.

4. Therapy

1) Chinese medicinal herbs

Referential prescription

Powder of Radix Rubiae combined with Decoction of Five Roots.

Chinese medicinal herbs commonly used

Radix Rehmanniae, Radix Scrophulariae, Cortex Moutan Radicis, Radix Paeoniae Rubra, Radix Rubiae, Radix Arnebiae seu Lithospermi, Herba Oldenlandiae Diffusae, Scolopendra, Agkistrodon Acutus, Rhizoma Imperatae.

Formulated preparation: Pill of Venenum Bufonis, 5-15 grains, po, bid (33 grains amount to 1 g roughly); Pill for Arousing Dissipation, 3-9 g, po, qd or bid; Pill of Western Calculus Bovis, 3 g, po, bid; Minor Golden Pellet, 0.6-1.2 g, po, bid.

Modification of herbs

Hectic fever and night sweat: add Radix Stellariae, Cortex Lycii Radicis, Plastrum Testudinis, Radix Oryzae Glutinosae.

Dizziness: add Fructus Lycii, Fructus Ligustri Lucidi, Flos Chrysanthemi (Alba).

Hemorrhage: add Rhizoma Anemarrhenae, Herba Ecliptae, Herba Agrimoniae.

Lymphadenectasis: add Spica Prunellae, Bulbus Cremastrae, Spina Gleditsiae, Concha Ostreae.

2) Acupuncture and moxibustion

Principal acupoints: LI11, LI4, BL40, SP10, SP6; reducing manipulation. Adjunct acupoints: BL23, KI3, KI6, SI36, BL18; invigorating manipulation.

VIII) Subacute and chronic encephalopathy or encephalitis (AIDS-dementia syndrome)

These are caused by the direct attack of HIV on CNS, and amount to 25-61.3% of damages of nervous system.

1. Principal symptoms and signs

Headache, dizziness, hypomnesia, disturbance in recognition, mental confusion, dementia, shortness of breath, palpitation, feebleness, weariness, even incontinence of urination and defecation; reddened or dim purple tongue with white and thin, or greasy coating; thready and uneven pulse.

2. Pathogenesis

Kidney is the origin of congenital constitution; brain is the residence of mental activity. Depletion of Kidney Essence and Marrow Sea brings about the hyperactivity of Yang, resulting in dizziness and headache. Hypomnesia, disturbance of recognition, mental confusion, dementia, and incontinence of urination and defecation are due to the blockage of Collaterals by Blood stasis or Phlegm agglutination, which is the outcome of Qi Asthenia. Shortness of breath, palpitation, weariness, and feebleness are manifestations of Qi and Blood deficiency.

3. Therapeutic principle

Nourish Kidney, strengthen Spleen, activate Blood, resolve Stasis, eliminate Phlegm, clear Apertures.

4. Therapy

1) Chinese medicinal herbs

Refern prescription

Seven Blessings Drink; Decoction for Opening Apertures and Activating Blood; Bolus for Treating Epilepsy.

Chinese medicinal herbs commonly used

Rhizoma Rehmanniae Praeparatae, Radix Ginseng, Radix

Angelicae Sinensis, Rhizoma Atractylodis Macrocephalae, Rhizoma Pinelliae, Arisaema cum Bile, Bombyx Batryticatus, Scolopendra, Semen Persicae, Flos Carthami, Rhizoma Acori Graminei.

Modification of herbs

Depletion of Kidney Essence: add Plastrum Testudinis, Colla Corii Asini.

Exuberance of Heart Fire, vexation, deep-coloured urine: add Plumula Nelumbinis, Rhizoma Coptidis.

Harassment of Phlegm-Fire interiorly: add Pill for Clearing Away Heart Fire and Expelling Phlegm, 3 g, po, bid.

Serious headache: add Buthus martensi, Ramulus Uncariae cum Uncis, Spica Prunellae.

Dizziness: add Fructus Lycii, Herba Ecliptae, Fructus Ligustri Lucidi.

Obvious shortness of breath and feebleness: add Radix Astragali seu Hedysari, Radix Codonopsis Pilosulae, Semen Ziziphi Spinosae, Radix Polygalae, Poria cum Ligno Hospite.

2) Acupuncture and moxibustion

Principal acupoints: GV20, ST40, LR3; reducing manipulation. Adjunct acupoints: BT23, KI3, ST36, SP6; invigorating manipulation.

III. TCM Measures for Health Protection

Various measures for health protection had been developed in ancient times and rich experiences had been accumulated by Chinese from generation to generation. Among them, acupuncture-moxibustion and Qigong are the most effective. According to results of current medical research, they may not only strengthen body resistance, but also improve or regulate human immunologic function. In view of the fact that AIDS is characterized by immune deficiency and no satisfactory drugs or vaccines have been prepared at present, we expect these measures will play an important role as adjuvant therapies of AIDS.

I) Acupuncture and Moxibustion

Ancient doctors had pointed out: "When CV4, CV6, GV4 and CV12 are cauterized frequently with moxa in healthy state, one may live a long life for more than one hundred years, even though eternal life is impossible". The effect of acupuncture and moxibustion in protecting health has also been confirmed by current clinical and experimental studies.

1. Methods of acupuncture and moxibustion for health protection

ST36, CV4 and CV6 are principal acupoints used for health protection; but each time ST36 must be selected with one of the other two acupoints alternately. ST36 may be manipulated independently. Such therapy is usually carried out 2-3 times per week.

Generally, ST36 is acupunctured with invigorating manipulation or weak stimulation. The needle is withdrawn after needling sensations have been obtained, or after that the acupoint is cauterized with moxa for 3 min.

CV4 and CV6 are cauterized with moxa-stick (mild moxibustion) for 3-5 min, until a tolerable warm or hot sensation is felt and flushing occurs at the local part.

2. Various methods of moxibustion for health protection

1) Cauterization of CV8 with moxa

CV8 belongs to Conception Vessel Meridian. Its principal therapeutic effects are warming and invigorating Primordial Yang, strengthening Spleen-Stomach, resuscitating, and consolidating the collapse of Primordial Energy. There are two methods for its cauterization.

① Ginger-partitioned moxibustion

Place a slice of fresh ginger (2-4 mm thick) on the navel. The ginger slice had been prickled with a needle to get small openings. Cauterize it with 3-5 moxa cones successively until a warm and comfortable sensation is perceived and local flushing occurs. Such manipulation should be performed every other day. Beware of scorching burn.

② Salt-partitioned moxibustion

Fill the navel fossa with fine, clean salt grains, then put a moxa cone on it. Cauterize CV8 with 3-5 moxa cones successively every other day. Matters needing attention are the same as ginger-partitioned moxibustion.

The above mentioned two methods may be used cooperatively.

2) Cauterization of ST36 with moxa

ST36 is the Sea Point of Stomach Meridian. Its therapeutic effects are invigorating and benefiting Spleen-Stomach, regulating and harmonizing Qi and Blood, strengthening body resistance, fostering Primordial Vitality, expelling pathogenic evil, and preventing disease.

Ignite a moxa stick, keeping it away from ST36 at a distance of about 3cm; cauterize ST36 for 10-15 min, until the local part becomes slightly flushed. Such moxibustion should be carried out every other day.

3) Cauterization of CV6 with moxa

CV6 belongs to Conception Vessel Meridian; its another name is Elixir Field (Dantian). Its therapeutic effects are fostering and invigorating Primordial Qi, benefiting Kidney, and consolidating Essence. There are two methods of CV6 moxibustion.

① Mild moxibustion

Refer to manipulations of mild moxibustion of ST36.

② Ginger-partitioned moxibustion

Let the patient lie supinely. Place a slice of fresh ginger (3-5mm thick) on CV6, which had been prickled with a needle to get several openings. Cauterize it with 3-10 moxa cones successively, which are of soya bean size or date-pit size. Such moxibustion should be carried out once every day, every other day, or every third day.

4) Cauterization of CV4 with moxa

In TCM, CV4 is also called Elixir Field (Dantian). It is the Meeting Point of Three Yin Meridians of the Foot and Conception Vessel Meridian, and the Accumulating Point of Small Intestine Meridian. Its therapeutic effects are warming Kidney, consolidating Essence, invigorating Qi, recuperating Yang, clearing and regulating Vital and Conception Vessel Meridians, rectifying Qi, and harmonizing Blood.

Mild moxibustion and ginger-partitioned moxibustion are often selected. Manipulations are the same as those mentioned in moxibustion of CV6.

5) Cauterization of GV14 with moxa

GV14 is the Meeting Point of Three Yang Meridians of the Hand and Foot and Governor Vessel Meridian. It governs all Yang Meridians and dominates the whole body. Its therapeutic effects are relieving Exterior, activating Yang, expelling Wind-Cold, sobering and tranquilizing the mind.

Mild moxibustion of GV14 is often selected. Manipulations are the same as those mentioned in mild moxibustion of ST36.

6) Cauterization of BL12 with moxa

BL12 is the Meeting Point of Governor Vessel Meridian and Taiyang Meridian of the Foot. Its therapeutic effects are ventilating Lung Qi, relieving Exterior, removing obstruction in Collaterals, expelling Wind, regulating and rectifying Qi mechanism.

Ginger-partitioned moxibustion is often selected; 10-20 moxa cones with a size of soya bean are burnt successively every day.

7) Cauterization of GV12 with moxa

GV12 belongs to Governor Vessel Meridian. Its therapeutic effects are communicating Yang, rectifying Qi, expelling Wind, abating fever, sobering and tranquilizing the mind, depressing the adverse flow of Qi, and stopping cough.

Mild moxibustion of GV12 is often selected.

8) Cauterization of KI16 with moxa

KI16 belongs to Taiyang Meridian of the Foot. Its therapeutic effects are ventilating and rectifying Lung Qi, benefiting Qi and replenishing deficiency.

Ginger-partitioned moxibustion of KI16 is often selected.

9) Cauterization of KI1 with moxa

KI1 is the Well Point of Shaoying Meridian of the Foot. Its therapeutic effects are tranquilizing the mind, clearing Apertures, replenishing and benefiting Kidney Essence, dispersing and regulating Liver Qi.

Let the patient lie pronely. Place a slice of fresh ginger (about 4 mm thick) on KI1, cauterize it with 5-10 moxa cones once every other day. The moxa cone is of the size of a soya bean.

In addition to methods mentioned above, CV12, SP6, BL23, GV4, LI11, GB34, etc., may also be cauterized with moxa. They may be selected or incorporated according to specific disease conditions.

The important thing of moxibustion for health protection lies in the perseverance of its practice. It may improve immunologic function, regulate physiologic activities, and reinforce the body resistance of patients suffering from AIDS or ARC.

II Qigong

Qigong is a kind of physicopsychic training which demands a full play of the trainee's intentional activity. In practising such exercise, mental and physical (breathing) activities are dynamically integrated, bringing about beneficial influences to one's health. It may tranquilize one's mind, correct one's emotional lability, reinforce one's body resistance, and promote the rehabilitation of one's disease by oneself. Current medical research has demonstrated that immunologic function may also be improved or regulated along with the practice of Qigong. Therefore, it is a good adjuvant therapy in the treatment of AIDS.

At the initial stage of undertaking Qigong, it would be best to consult a specialist in this domain, thereby deviations or errors in practice and side effects may be avoided. The guarantee of obtaining success in Qigong lies in one's confidence and perseverance. "Go fishing for three days and dry the nets for two" will certainly be of no help.

Several common practices of Qigong are recommended as follows:

1. Exercise for Psychosomatic Relaxation and Tranquilization

1) Posture: Sitting, standing, or lying.

2) Respiration: Natural breathing at the beginning, then change it into abdominal breathing gradually.

3) Intentional focus: Concentrate intention on one's own Elixir Field or on an exterior object.

4) Exercising method: Having assumed a certain posture, close one's eyes slightly, tranquilize one's mind, regulate one's

respiration, then relax oneself. Details of self-relaxation in a respiratory cycle are as follows: Relax oneself from one's head to one's Elixir Field and from the shoulder to the elbow, cooperating with one expiration. After one natural inspiration, relax oneself from Elixir Field to the sacrum-coxa region and from two elbows to both hands, cooperating with another expiration. Then after another natural inspiration, relax oneself from the sacrum-coxa region to both centres of one's soles, coorperating with one expiration. Within one respiratory cycle, mutter "Tranquility" silently during inspiration, mutter "Relaxation" silently during expiration.

5) Ending of this exercise: Imagine Respiratory Qi from various parts of one's body is gathering slowly toward one's Elixir Field. At this moment, a beginner may put the centre of one palm on his (her) navel, keeping the centre of the other palm piled up on the dorsum of the former hand. Then assume the navel as a centre, move both hands toward the left side of the navel and push them around it slowly and circularly for 20-30 cycles, increasing the radius gradually until they reach the precordial region. Stop such pushing around. After a little while, move both hands from the precordial region to the right side and push them around the navel slowly and circularly along an opposite direction, decreasing the radius gradually. The number of circles revolved should be equal to that performed previously. Stop pushing around, keep both hands at the navel. Thereafter, rub two hands gently, open both eyes, move one's body, and finish this exercise.

2. Exercise for Nourishing the Interior

1) Posture: Lying on one's side or sitting upright mostly; or lying pronely, or sitting with crossed legs.

2) Respiration: Change natural respiration into abdominal or inverse respiration. When the exerciser becomes fairly skilled

in such breathing, try to practise "Respiration with intermittent pausing"; i.e. in the course of transnasal abdominal respiration, stop the respiratory movement for a little while after each respiratory cycle, cooperated with silent muttering of words and expressions.

Details of "Respiration with intermittent pausing" are as follows: During inspiration, prop the palate softly with the lingual tip, mutter the first word silently; meanwhile lead the inspired Qi into one's Elixir Field, swelling the lower abdomen slowly, thereafter begin the expiration. During expiration, prop the inner surface of lower incisor teeth with the lingual tip, mutter the second word silently; meanwhile shrink the lower abdomen slowly. After expiration, stop the respiratory movement naturally, the tongue proper and the abdomen remain motionless, and mutter silently the third word. Such a sequence of inspiration-expiration-pausing is repeated again and again. The duration of respiratory pausing should be lengthened gradually by adding the number of words silently muttered, for instance, from 3 to 7 or 8. Self suggestion should be implicated in words and expressions silently muttered, such as "Relaxation is good", "Relaxation is very good", "Relaxation is good for my health", etc.

3) Intentional focus: Concentrate intention on one's own Elixir Field; or on an exterior object at the beginning, then shift the intentional focus to Elixir Field.

4) Exercising method: Assume a posture mentioned previously. Practise the Exercise for Psychosomatic Relaxation and Tranquilization for 3-5 min; thereafter begin the Exercise for Nourishing the Interior.

5) Ending of this exercise: Refer to descriptions in Exercise for Psychosomatic Relaxation and Tranquilization.

3. Exercise of Standing like a Stake

1) Posture: There are many postures recommended for practising this kind of exercise. Generally, a beginner starts from a natural standing posture.

① Standing like a stake while both hands assuming a posture of pressing a ball. The intensity of sustaining strength is greater than that in natural standing, but muscles should be relaxed.

② Standing like a stake while both arms assuming a posture of circular embracing. Stand naturally, raise both arms to the level of breasts before the chest with palms facing inwardly and fingers slightly crooked and separated from each other. Finger tips of both hands oppose each other and they are at a distance of about two fists. The two arms are flexed as if they are embracing a big tree. Nevertheless, strength is exerted both toward the exterior and toward the interior. The former accounts for 30%, the latter 70%, and they are exerted alternately.

2) Respiration: Principally natural breathing, practise abdominal respiration step by step.

3) Intentional focus: Concentrate intention on an exterior object, looking horizontally.

4) Exercising method: Assume an appropriate posture. Practise Exercise for Psychosomatic Relaxation and Tranquilization for 3-5 min. Close one's eyes loosely, regulate one's breathing, tranquilize one's mind, and sink Qi into one's Elixir Field. Thereafter lead Qi to Elixir Field during inspiration, stop breathing for a little while. Then lead Qi from Elixir Field to centres of both feet. At this moment, try to clutch the ground with both feet gently, imagine one's body being like an old pine tree towering erect. Practise this exercise perseverantly. With the passing of time, one may feel he (she) is full of vigor.

5) Ending of this exercise: Refer to descriptions in Exercise for Psychosomatic Relaxation and Tranquilization.

4. Inducive Exercise

1) Inducement of relaxation

Assume an appropriate posture. Imagine that oneself is situated in a quiet, peaceful, and comfortable environment, breathing fresh air in pleasant weather, and is full of care-free, joyous and ease temper. After one's mood has been calmed, imagine relaxation begins from one's head, neck, trunk, and then the four limbs gradually. Repeat such intentional activity successively for several times.

2) Inducement of respiration

In regulating respiratory movement, put forth one's strength slightly in the action of inspiration to lengthen its duration, assisted by intentional force. This is an easy way to achieve the required respiratory pattern.

3) Inducement of intentional focus

When an exerciser cannot concentrate his (her) intention on his (her) Elixir Field due to the interference of frequent distracting thoughts, he (she) may put both hands on the lower abdomen to warm it. Warm and comfortable sensation contribute to the elimination of distracting thoughts and the concentration of intentional focus.

4) Therapeutic induction

When the interference of distracting thoughts is mitigated and the relaxation of the whole body is achieved, one may begin to practise therapeutic induction. For instance, patients suffering from hypertension may assume a standing posture, imagine a continuous drizzle is falling down on their bodies and the rain-water is flowing downwards from their heads to their trunks and extremities. Through such induction, the blood pressure may be reduced and the symptom of top-heavy may be alleviated or even eliminated.

Patients suffering from AIDS may try such therapeutic induction according to their disease conditions.

IV. Dietotherapy

In China, foods and drugs are of the same origin. Many foods may be used as prophylactic, roborant, or therapeutic drugs, since they are nutrients and medicines at the same time. Rich experiences have been accumulated in taking such foods from generation to generation. Consequently, it is self evident that dietotherapy is a precious treasure of TCM.

I) Dietotherapeutic principles in treating AIDS

1. Proper dietary regimen

The basic principle of dietary regimen is to take a suitable amount but various kinds of foods and drinks at fixed times. Overeating, overfasting, and taking diets at irregular time will certainly do harm to Spleen-Stomach, while food preference may lead to excess or deficiency of essential nutrient elements, and the impairment of health.

Patients suffering from AIDS are listless, despondent, and sluggish generally; their dietary regimens are violated due to physical torture and mental distress. It is evident that such violation is extremely disadvantageous to their convalescence, and the establishment of proper dietary regimen is of great importance.

2. Property and compatibility of diets

Property of diets in TCM indicates their Four Natures, Five Tastes, as well as their other attributes, for instance lifting, lowering, floating, and sinking; and Meridian tropism.

1) Four Natures

These indicate the cold, hot, warm, and cool natures of diets.

Generally speaking, cool and cold diets may clear away Heat, purge Fire, and resolve Toxin; warm and hot diets may warm Yang and disperse Cold. There are also diets of bland nature, which may be taken by patients suffering from either Hot or Cold Syndrome

2) Five Tastes

These indicate sour, bitter, sweet, acrid, and salty tastes. In fact, there is another taste, namely insipidness. According to TCM, diets of sour taste are astringent; they may refrain and consolidate. Diets of bitter taste may dry Wetness, clear away Heat, and purge Sthenia. Diets of sweet taste may nourish the body, relax spasm, and harmonize various diet natures and tastes. Diets of acrid taste may induce diaphoresis, activate Qi, and stop pain. Diets of salty taste may soften and resolve hard masses and nodules; in addition, they may also bring about moistening, nourishing, and retrieving effects.

According to TCM, there are close relations between Five Solid Viscera and Five Tastes: The acrid taste enters Lung, the sweet taste enters Spleen, the bitter taste enters Heart, the sour taste enters Liver, the salty taste enters Kidney.

Foods like drugs, after having been taken, give rise to various pharmacologic effects, such as lifting, lowering, floating, and sinking. Therefore, a proper selection and compatibility of foods and drinks are essential to the health protection of asthenic patients, especially those suffering from AIDS.

3. Diets should not be greasy

It is held by TCM that overeating of greasy and strongly flavoured diets is harmful to Spleen-Stomach or one's health.

Patients suffering from AIDS are deficient in Kidney Essence, Qi, and Blood. Under these circumstances, pathologic changes of Asthenia are liable to be transformed into Heat or Wind, thereby resulting in Blood activation, Blood stasis, or Phlegm stagnation. For instance, fat meat, wine, or greasy, pungent foods contribute to the production and accumulation of Wetness and Phlegm, upward hyperactivity of Liver Yang, stirring of Liver Wind, and the arising of carbuncles, ulcers, or other pyogenic infections. All these variations accelerate the deterioration of AIDS.

Thus, to patients suffering from AIDS, the following diets are recommended:

Staple food: Rice, wheat, or cereals other than rice and wheat, such as millets, beans, etc.

Non-staple food: Vegetables, bean products, supplemented by lean meat, soft-shelled turtle, freshwater fish, etc.

II) Edibles recommended to patients suffering from AIDS

1. Rhizoma Dioscoreae

Nature: bland; Taste: sweet.

Effects: Strengthen Spleen, invigorate Lung, consolidate Kidney, benefit Essence.

Indications: Anorexia, dyspepsia, diarrhea, and cough due to consumptive diseases.

Cooking method: Rhizoma Dioscoreae may be cooked with an appropriate amount of rice to make gruel.

2. Fructus Ziziphi Jujubae

Nature: warm; Taste: sweet.

Effects: Invigorate Middle Energizer, benefit Qi, nourish Blood, tranquilize the mind.

Indications: Lassitude, feebleness, poor appetite, loose stool, Blood Asthenia with sallow complexion.

Cooking method: Fructus Ziziphi Jujubae may be cooked with Semen Phaseoli to make gruel.

3. Auricularia auricula

Nature: bland; Taste: sweet.

Effects: Moisten dryness, facilitate intestine, cool Blood, stop bleeding.

Indications: Hemorrhagic tendency.

Cooking method: Auricularia auricula may be stewed with an appropriate amount of sugar.

4. Fructus Mume

Nature: bland; Taste: sour and astringent.

Effects: Promote the production of body fluids, quench thirst, astringe Lung, stop cough, diarrhea and bleeding.

Indications: Dry cough with little phlegm, even hemoptysis; diarrhea.

Cooking method: In case of dry cough with little phlegm or even hemoptysis, cook Fructus Mume with an appropriate amount of Bulbus Lilii to make gruel. In case of diarrhea, cook Fructus Mume with Semen Coicis and sugar to make gruel.

5. Tremella fuciformis

Nature: bland; Taste: sweet, insipid.

Effects: Nourish Yin, moisten Lung, benefit Stomach, promote the production of body fluids.

Indications: Dry cough with little phlegm, dry mouth and throat, even epistaxis, hemoptysis.

Cooking method: Tremella fuciformis may be stewed with an appropriate amount of sugar.

6. Gracilaria verrucosa

Nature: cold; Taste: sweet and salty.

Effects: Clear away Heat, soften hard masses, resolve Phlegm.

Indications: Lymphadenectasis accompanied with fever.

Cooking method: Gracilaria verrucosa may be taken as non-staple foodstuffs.

7. Arillus Longan

Nature: warm; Taste: sweet.

Effects: Benefit Heart-Spleen, replenish Qi and Blood, tranquilize the mind.

Indications: Emaciation, weakness, insomnia, amnesia, palpitation due to fright, severe palpitation.

Cooking method: Arillus Longan may be taken as fruits or desserts. It may also be stewed with Fructus Ziziphi Jujubae.

Contraindications: Manifestations caused by hyperactivity of Fire resulting from Yin deficiency, such as fever, night sweat, etc.

8. Colocasia esculenta

Nature: bland; Taste: sweet and acrid.

Effects: Resolve scrofula, disperse stagnation.

Indications: Lymphadenectasis.

Cooking method: Colocasia esculenta may be cooked as staple food or non-staple food.

9. Bulbus Lilii

Nature: slightly cold; Taste: sweet and insipid.

Effects: Moisten Lung, stop cough, clear away Heart Fire, tranquilize the mind.

Indications: Dry cough, even hemoptysis due to Lung Dryness; low fever, asthenic vexation.

Cooking method: Bulbus Lilii may be cooked with an appropriate amount of crystal sugar.

10. Colla Corii Asini

Nature: bland; Taste: sweet.

Effects: Nourish Yin and Blood, invigorate Lung, moisten Dryness, stop bleeding.

Indications: Anemia or accompanied with loss of blood.

Cooking method: Colla Corii Asini may be stewed with crystal sugar.

11. Semen Phaseoli

Nature: bland; Taste: sweet and sour.

Effects: Promote diuresis, eliminate edema, clear away Heat, resolve Toxin.

Indications: Eczema, cutaneous pyogenic infection or ulceration.

Cooking method: Semen Phaseoli may be cooked to make gruel.

12. Semen Euryales

Nature: bland; Taste: sweet and astringent.

Effects: Strengthen Spleen, stop diarrhea, consolidate Kidney, astringe Essence.

Indications: Chronic diarrhea, aching of the waist, nocturnal emission.

Cooking method: Semen Euryales may be cooked alone to make gruel; or cooked with Semen Nelumbinis and Semen Coicis to make gruel.

13. Tortoise meat

Nature: bland; Taste: sweet and salty.

Effects: Benefit Yin, replenish Blood.

Indications: Hectic fever, protracted cough, hemoptysis, aching of the waist, atrophic debility of bones.

Cooking method: Tortoise meat may be stewed with condiments.

14. Thallus Laminariae seu Eckloniae

Nature: cold; Taste: salty.

Effects: Soften hard masses, promote diuresis.

Indications: Lymphadenectasis.

Cooking method: Thallus Laminariae seu Eckloniae may be cooked as non-staple foodstuffs.

15. Juglandis Regiae

Nature: warm; Taste: sweet.

Effects: Invigorate Kidney, warm lung, relieve dyspnea,

moisten Intestine.

Indications: Cough and dyspnea caused by depletion of both Lung and Kidney.

Cooking method: Juglandis Regiae may be stir-fried until it is done.

Contraindications: Cough due to Yin Asthenia, diarrhea, loose stool.

16. Poria coccos

Nature: bland; Taste: sweet and insipid.

Effects: Strengthen Spleen, eliminate Wetness, relieve mental distress, tranquilize the mind. According to results of pharmacologic studies, it is also an anticarcinogen and may improve the immunologic function.

Indications: Kaposi's sarcoma, lymphadenectasis, chronic diarrhea, etc.

Cooking method: Poria coccos may be cooked with Semen Coicis, Rhizoma Dioscoreae to make gruel.

17. Semen Dolichoris

Nature: bland; Taste: sweet.

Effects: Strengthen Spleen, harmonize Middle Energizer, relieve Summer-Heat, eliminate Wetness. Current pharmacologic studies have demonstrated it is an anticancer and antiviral agent, and it may stimulate the immunologic function.

Indications: Asthenic Syndromes.

Cooking method: Cooked as staple or non-staple food.

18. Cormus Eleocharis Dulcis

Nature: cold; Taste: sweet.

Effects: Clear away Heat, resolve phlegm, eliminate stagnation.

Indications: Fever, cough, swelling and pain of the throat.

Cooking method: Cormus Eleocharis Dulcis may be eaten raw (peeled), or cooked as staple or non-staple.

19. Lentinus edodes

Nature: bland; Taste: sweet.

Effects: Invigorate Qi, benefit Stomach. It is also an anticancer and antiviral agent, and may improve the immunologic function.

Indications: Asthenic Syndromes.

Cooking method: Lentinus edodes may be cooked as non-staple food. Nature: bland; Taste: sweet and astringent.

20. Semen Nelembinis

Effects: Nourish Heart, benefit Kidney, invigorate Spleen, astringe Intestine.

Indications: Diarrhea, dysentery, dreaminess, nocturnal emission, aching of the waist, etc.

Cooking method: Semen Nelumbinis may be cooked with Semen Euryales, Poris coccos, Semen Coicis, and Semen Dolichoris to make gruel.

21. Laminaria japonica

Nature: cold; Taste: salty.

Effects: Soften hard masses, resolve Phlegm, promote diuresis, purge Heat.

Indications: Lymphadenectasis.

Cooking method: Laminaria japonica may be cooked as non-staple food.

22. Rhopilema esculentum

Nature: bland; Taste: salty.

Effects: Clear away Heat, resolve Phlegm, eliminate stagnation, moisten Intestine.

Indications: Cough with phlegm, dyspnea, hypochondriac lump, feeling of distension and fullness of the abdomen, constipation with dry stool.

Cooking method: Rhopilema esculentum may be cooked or eaten raw as non-staple food.

23. Sargassum tortile or S. enerve

Nature: cold; Taste: salty.

Effects: Soften hard masses, resolve Phlegm, promote diuresis, purge Heat.

Indications: Lymphadenectasis.

Cooking method: Sargassum tortile may be cooked as non-staple food.

24. Sea Cucumber

Nature: warm; Taste: sweet and salty.

Effects: Invigorate Kidney, benefit Essence, nourish Blood, moisten Dryness.

Indications: Manifestations of depletion of Essence and Blood, such as dizziness, feebleness, aching of the waist, nocturnal emission, etc.

Cooking method: Sea Cucumber may be cooked as non-staple food.

25. Duck meat

Nature: bland; Taste: sweet and salty.

Effects: Foster Stomach, nourish Yin, promote diuresis, eliminate edema.

Indications: Hectic fever, cough, bodily Asthenia.

Cooking method: Duck meat is cooked as non-staple food.

26. Hemerocallis Flava

Nature: bland; Taste: sweet.

Effects: Nourish Blood, calm Liver, promote diuresis, eliminate edema.

Indications: Dizziness, tinnitus, sore throat, palpitation, hemorrhage, cutaneous pyogenic infections.

Cooking method: Hemerocallis Flava may be cooked as non-staple food.

27. Semen Phaseoli Radiatus

Nature: cool; Taste: sweet.

Effects: Clear away Heat, resolve Toxin, relieve Summer-Heat, promote diuresis.

Indications: Fever, polydipsia, diarrhea, dysentery, eczema, herpes, etc.

Cooking method: Semen Phaseoli Radiatus may be cooked to make gruel.

28. Cooked and dried Mussel

Nature: warm; Taste: salty.

Effects: Invigorate Liver-Kidney, benefit Essence and Blood, resolve goiter and tumour.

Indications: Manifestations of Yin Asthenia of Liver-Kidney, such as consumptive state, emaciation, hectic fever, night sweat, lymphadenectasis.

Cooking method: Mussel may be cooked as non-staple food.

29. Hydnum erinaceus

Nature: bland; Taste: sweet.

Effects: Replenish Asthenia, stimulate appetite. It may also improve immunologic function.

Indications: Leukopenia, Kaposi's sarcoma.

Cooking method: Hydnum erinaceus may be cooked as non-staple food.

30. Semen Sojae Nigrum

Nature: bland; Taste: sweet.

Effects: Activate Blood, promote diuresis, expel Wind, resolve Toxin.

Indications: Cutaneous pyogenic infections.

Cooking method: Semen Sojae Nigrum may be cooked to make gruel or staple food.

31. Honey

Nature: bland; Taste: sweet.

Effects: Invigorate Middle Energizer, moisten Dryness, relieve pain, resolve Toxin.

Indications: Cough due to Lung Dryness, ulcerative stomatitis, etc.

Contraindications: Diarrhea, loose stool.

32. Coturnix coturnix japonica

Nature: warm; Taste: sweet.

Effects: Invigorate Five Solid Viscera, benefit Middle Energizer, strengthen Tendons and Bones, clear away Wetness-Heat.

Indications: Asthenia of Spleen-Stomach, anorexia, aching of Tendons and Bones, feebleness, weariness, etc.

Cooking method: Coturnix coturnix japonica may be cooked asnon-staple food.

33. Semen Coicis

Nature: cool; Taste: sweet and insipid.

Effects: Strengthen Spleen, invigorate Lung, clear away and eliminate Wetness-Heat. It is also an anticancer and antiviral agent.

Indications: Diarrhea, eczema, etc.

Cooking method: Semen Coicis may be cooked with Poria coccos, Semen Dolichoris, Semen Phaseoli, etc. , to make gruel.

34. Meat of soft-shelled turtle

Nature: bland; Taste: sweet.

Effects: Nourish Yin, cool Blood.

Indications: Manifestations of Yin Asthenia of Liver-Kidney, such as aching of the waist, weakness of knees, insomnia, dreaminess, night sweat, tuberculosis, etc.

Cooking method: Meat of soft-shelled turtle may be cooked as non-staple foodstuff.

Section 6. Seeking for Effective Agents from Chinese Herbal Medicines to Treat AIDS

Since no effective drugs or vaccines are available, many medical scientists lay their hopes on TCM. As a matter of fact, researches in this domain have been energetically carried out in America, Japan, and other countries. Here, we recommend several Chinese herbal medicines and prescriptions which are worthy of further exploration.

I. Prescriptions for the Prophylaxis and Treatment of AIDS

1. Bolus for Regulating Middle Energizer or Decoction of Radix Ginseng (cited from *Treatise on Exogenous Febrile Diseases*).

Composition: Radix Ginseng 6 g, Rhizoma Zingiberis (dried) 9 g, Rhizoma Atractylodis Macrocephalae 9 g, Radix Glycyrrhizae (fried with liquid adjuvants) 9 g.

Such bolus or decoction had been transformed into a Dissoluble Granule Preparation by Hanedamasao, Tokyo Medical College, and such preparation was administered to 4 hemophiliacs with positive HIV antibody. The dosage was 2.5 g/day. Results indicated that it may increase the decreasing amount of T helper cell (TH), increase the amount of cells which may suppress the recombination of HIV, and increase the amount of natural killer cell obviously. It may inhibit the onset of AIDS in asymptomatic HIV carrier and ARC, and ameliorate the immunologic function in hemophiliacs with negative HIV antibody.

2. Minor Decoction of Radix Bupleuri (Cited from *Treatise on Exogenous Febrile Diseases*).

Composition: Radix Bupleuri 12 g, Radix Scutellariae 9 g, Radix Ginseng 3 g, Rhizoma Pinelliae 9 g, Radix Glycyrrhizae Praeparata 3 g, Rhizoma Zingiberis Recens 9 g, Fructus Ziziphi Jujubae 4 pieces.

This decoction may promote the production of polyclonal antibody and antibody of sheep erythrocyte caused by poke weed mitogen in vitro, improve the hypofunctional immune state caused by the administration of adrenocortical steroids and cyclophosphamide, and restore the immunosuppressive state of macrophage caused by carrageenin. When extracts of Radix Bupleuri and Radix Glycyrrhizae are used alone, the production of antibody is also increased. Radix Bupleuri itself may activate macrophage, and promote the production of interleukin-1 (IL-1). Interleukin-1 may increase the production of interleukin-2 (IL-2) which is originated from T lymphocytes; and while promoting the proliferation and differentiation of T lymphocytes, IL-1 may also promote the proliferation and differentiation of B lymphocytes with a tendency of transforming them into antibody producing cells afterwards. Consequently, the main effect of Minor Decoction of Radix Bupleuri or its principal ingredients is to act on macrophage and promote the production of antibody. Hanedamasao et al. held Minor Decoction of Radix Bupleuri may activate immunologic function, and such effect is associated with the activation of T suppressor cell and T helper cell. A Dissoluble Granule Preparation of this decoction was administered to 5 hemophiliacs with positive HIV antibody; the dosage was 4.5

g/day. Results indicated that the decreasing amount of T helper lymphocytes is increased.

3. Radix Puerariae Decoction (cited from *Treatise on Exogenous Febrile Diseases*).

Composition: Ramulus Cinnamomi 9 g, Radix Paeoniae Alba 9 g, Radix Glycyrrhizae 6 g, Rhizoma Zingiberis Recens 9 g, Fructus Ziziphi Jujubae 4 pieces, Radix Puerariae 10 g, Herba Ephedrae 6 g.

It has been demonstrated that this prescription may promote the production of antibody, presumably due to the action on macrophage by some ingredients in Radix Puerariae, Radix Glycyrrhizae, Radix Paeoniae Alba, or Rhizoma Zingiberis Recens. Further researches deserve to be carried out.

4. Polyporus Umbellatus Decoction (cited from *Treatise on Exogenovs Febrile Diseases*).

Composition: Polyporus Umbellatus 9 g, Rhizoma Alismatis 9 g, Poria coccos 9 g, Talcum 9 g, Colla Corii Asini 9 g.

This decoction may strengthen immunologic function and invigorate the phagocytic function of macrophage. Therefore, it may be used in the prophylaxis and treatment of AIDS on probation.

In addition, there are other prescriptions which may improve immunologic function, such as Decoction of Four Noble Drugs, Decoction of Four Drugs, Radix Astragali seu Hedysari Decoction for Invigorating Middle Energizer, Bolus (or Decoction) of Six Drugs Including Radix Rehmanniae, Bolus for Invigorating Middle Energizer and Benefiting Qi, Bolus for Restoring the Left Kidney, Pill of Six Miraculous Drugs, Jade Screen Powder, Powder for Restoring Pulse Beat, etc.

II. Chinese Medicinal Herbs for the Prophylaxis and Treatment of AIDS

1. Radix Glycyrrhizae

It had been observed experimentally in vitro that a solution with 0.5 mmg/mml of Glycyrrhizin may inhibit the multiplication of HIV to an extent of more than 98% in cells infected; and a solution with 0.125 mmg/mml of Glycyrrhizin may inhibit the multiplication of HIV to an extent of 50%. These results signify that Radix Glycyrrhizae may be effective in blocking the deterioration of physical condition of asymptomatic HIV carriers. At present, it has been demonstrated that Glycyrrhizin may induce the production of interferon, invigorate the activity of natural killer cell, and inhibit the multiplication of varicella-zoster virus.

2. Cordyceps Sinensis

Cordyceps Sinensis is a Chinese medicinal herb with tonifying effect. It had been shown that polysaccharides recovered from Cordyceps Sinensis possess a variety of pharmacologic and immunologic properties. When a dosage of 1-3 g, tid, was administered to patients suffering from tumor who are receiving chemotherapy, phagocytic activity was activated. Experimental research had demonstrated that polysaccharides of Cordyceps Sinensis may evidently stimulate the phagocytic activity of macrophage both in abdominal cavity and in reticuloendothelial system; the transformation of lymphocytes is also accelerated to a certain degree. Thus, it is reasonable to use Cordyceps Sinensis as an immunopotentiator in the prophylaxis and treatment of AIDS.

3. Lentinus edodes

Japanese medical workers had reported that after the infusion of Lentinan, decrease of HIV antibody occurred in 2 patients; in addition, during such infusion, induction or increase of interferon occurred in male patients. It was inferred that Lentinus edodes may improve the immunologic state and may be effective in treating patients suffering from AIDS, ARC, and HIV carriers. Experimental studies had demonstrated Lentinan may restore the phagocytic function of macrophage in the abdominal cavity of mice impaired by hydrocortisone, restore the T lymphocyte percentage in peripheral blood decreased by hydrocortisone, and restore the phagocytic function of reticuloendothelial system in mice impaired by hydroprednisone acetate. It may also restore the inhibition of delayed hypersensitivity caused by cyclophosphamide. Besides, it may evidently promote the transformation of mouse lymphocyte induced by ConA, and PHA. Therefore, it is a restoring agent of T helper cells.

4. Radix Arnebiae seu Lithospermi

In TCM, this Chinese medicinal herb is used to prevent and treat measles. Screening tests had confirmed that only its polysaccharides are effective in blocking the multiplication of HSV-1 in vitro, while its fat-soluble ingredients are ineffective. Clinically, decoction of Radix Arnebiae seu Lithospermi and its eye drops are useful in the treatment of herpes simplex keratitis.

5. Polystictus versicolor

Proteoglycans and various kinds of amino acids of Polystictus versicolor may inhibit tumorigenesis of various kinds in animal models. Abdominal administration of this drug in mice increase their weight of thymus and spleen, and activate their macrophages to kill tumor cells. These suggest Polystictus versicolor may strengthen the immunologic function.

6. Poria coccos

Polysaccharides extracted from Poria coccos may resist tumorigenesis. Carboxymethyl polysaccharide of Poria coccos prepared through a semi-synthetic technology of liquid-solid phasic oscillation, is effective not only in resisting tumorigenesis and improving the function of T lymphocytes and macrophages, but also in stimulating the activity of three kinds of natural killer cells evidently in old-aged mice, or in those whose function has been inhibited by cycloposphamide and tumor.

7. Polyporus Umbellatus

Extracts of Polyporus Umbellatus may invigorate the immunologic function of mice, keep the activity of mononuclear macrophage system in normal state, and stimulate the vitality of acid phosphatase in mononuclear macrophage in the abdominal cavity of mice, thereby strengthen their phagocytic function. Such extracts may also inhibit the growth of transplanted sarcoma (S180) in mice with comparatively remarkable efficacy. Polysaccharides obtained from Polyporus Umbellatus are more effective than those obtained from Japanese homogenous species, hence their dosage is smaller.

8. Ganoderma Lucidum

There are many active ingredients in Ganoderma Lucidum, demonstrated to be effective in strengthening human immunologic function. They may increase the phagocytic ratio of macrophage, the percentage of T lymphocytes, and the level of antibody; moreover, they are bactericides. Therefore, Ganoderma Lucidum plays an important role in the protecting cellular immunity.

9. Gynostemma Pentaphy Lum (Thumb) mak

Various kinds of saponin ingredients had been separated from this drug; among them, ginsenoside Rb1, Rb3, Rd, etc. had been identified. Therefore, it may be used as a substitute for Radix Ginseng. Current data have indicated that Dissoluble Granule Preparation of Radix Ginseng is effective in treating AIDS to a certain extent.

It had also been demonstrated that this drug may evidently enhance the titer of hemagglutinative antibody in mice and strengthen their delayed hypersensitivity, thereby improve their immunocompetence. Other experimental studies indicated total saponins of this drug may inhibit the growth of solid tumor (S180) in mice, and kill S180 cells directly in vitro. Consequently, this Chinese medicinal herb may be used as an immunopotentiator or as an agent protecting the body against exogenous infection or tumorigenesis.

10. Actinidia Chinensis Planch

Polysaccharides extracted from its root had been found to be effective in the following aspects: Inhibition of experimental tumorigenesis, invigoration of the activity of natural killer cell, increase of the percentage of phagocytes in abdominal cavity and their phagocytic index, restoration of the delayed hypersensitivity depressed by cyclophosphamide, and remarkable enhancement of body resistance to certain pathogenic bacteria.

11. Radix Ginseng

Recent studies have demonstrated that Radix Ginseng may improve the state of health, resist the invasion of noxious factors, relieve fatigue, stimulate appetite, promote the function of male gonad, and accelerate hematopoiesis. It had also been observed that Prostil, a preparation containing various glucosides separated from Radix Ginseng, may promote the synthesis of DNA, RNA, protein (including immunoglobin), and lipid. It may also promote the cell division of bone marrow, hence numbers of RBC and WBC tend to increase.

12. Radix Acanthopanacis Senticosi

Effects of Radix Acanthopanacis Senticosi are similar to those of Radix Ginseng. Experimental studies of immunologic function have indicated it may evidently invigorate the phagocytic function of cells coming from inflammatory exudations in guinea pigs. In research of phagocytic function of the reticuloendothelial system in mice, along with the increase of dosage, Radix Acanthopanacis Senticosi may remarkably increase the clearance index of carbon particles injected through their caudal veins. In mice, the E rosette forming rate is raised by 1.2-1.8 times after the administration of this drug. Clinically, it may reinforce the body to resist nonspecific harmful stimulants, such as fatigue, hypoxia, cold, etc. Current data have proved that the decrease of peripheral WBC amount caused by cyclophosphamide may be prevented by the administration of Radix Acanthopanacis Senticosi.

III. Chinese Medicinal Herbs Promoting Lymphocyte Transformation and Invigorating Cellular Immunologic Function

Radix Astragali seu Hedysari, Radix Codonopsis Pilosulae, Ganoderma Lucidum seu Japonicum, Radix Ginseng, Rhizoma Polygonati, Radix Rehmanniae, Cornu Cervi Pantotrichum, Herba Epimedii, Rhizoma Curculiginis, Fructus Psoraleae, Semen Cuscutae, Herba Cynomorii, Cortex Phellodendri, Fungus Tremellae, Radix Paeoniae Alba, Fructus Lycii, Fructus Ligustri Lucidi, Ramulus Loranthi, Radix Polygoni Multiflori, Radix Paeoniae Rubra, Radix Angelicae Sinensis, Colla Corii Asini, Radix Phytotaccae, Caulis Spatholobi, Fructus Mori, Herba Taraxaci, Radix Bupleuri, Rhizoma Coptidis, Radix Scutellariae, Flos Lonicerae, Semen Coicis, Rhizoma Polygonati Odorati, Rhizoma Dioscoreae, Radix Glycycrrhizae, Radix Acanthopanacis Senticosi, Lentinus edodes, Polyporus, Umbellatus.

IV. Chinese Medicinal Herbs Inducing the Production of Interferon or Promoting the Induction of Interferon

Radix Astragali seu Hedysari, Radix Glycyrrhizae, Radix Ginseng, Lentinus edodes, Radix Acanthopanacis Senticosi, Radix Angelicae Dahuricae, Rhizoma Gastrodiae, Radix Stephaniae Tetrandrae, Rhizoma Ligustici Chuanxiong, Radix Sophorae Subprostratae, Radix Angelicae Sinensis, Radix Sophorae Flavescentis, Rhizoma Atractylodis Macrocephalae, Radix Bupleuri, Rhizoma Pinelliae, Rhizoma Cimicifugae, Radix Asparagi, Radix et Rhizoma Rhei, Flos Lonicerae, Radix Scutellariae, Flos Carthami, Herba Artemisiae Chinghao, Cortex Mori Radicis.

V. Chinese Medicinal Herbs Improving Phagocytic Function of Phagocytes

Radix Astragali seu Hedysari, Radix Codonopsis Pilosulae, Radix Giseng, Ganoderma Lucidum seu Japonicum, Radix Angelicae Sinensis, Rhizoma Atractylodis Macrocephalae, Rhizoma Dioscoreae, Herba Epimedii, Fructus Psoraleae, Cortex Phellodendri, Cortex Eucommiae, Herba Houttuyniae, Herba Oldenlandiae Diffusae, Indigo Naturalis, Rhizoma Coptidis, Radix Scutallariae, Flos Lonicerae, Folium Isatidis, Polyporus Umbellatus, Flos Daturae, Radix Acanthopanacis Senticosi, Radix Salviae Miltiorrhizae, Flos Carthami, Poria coccos, Cordyceps Sinensis, Herba Elsholtziae seu Moslae.

VI. Chinese Medicinal Herbs Promoting the Production of Antibody and Invigorating Humoral Immunologic Function

Radix Astragali seu Hedysari, Radix Ginseng, Rhizoma Polygonati, Radix Aconiti Praeparata, Radix Acanthopanacis Senticosi, Semen Cuscutae, Rhizoma Curculiginis, Cortex Cinnamomi, Herba Cynomorii, Radix Scrophulariae, Carapax Trionycis, Radix Asparagi, Radix Ophiopogonis, Fructus Ligustri Lucidi, Fructus Corni, Venenum Bufonis, Rhizoma Zingiberis Recens, Bulbus Allii, Semen Coicis, Radix Salviae Miltiorrhizae, Poria coccos, Polyporus Umbellatus.

Section 7. Requirements in the Treatment of AIDS with TCM and Its Specific Utilization

Since the first case of AIDS was reported, 10 years have passed. During this period, medical scholars all over the world have payed much attention to the significance of TCM in the prophylaxis and treatment of AIDS. Although there were no disease named AIDS and no special treatise dealing with AIDS in TCM history, related manuscripts about similar characteristic syndromes and their diagno-therapeutic methods may be noticed sporadically in many medical books. In order to deepen our understanding of the theories of TCM and to apply TCM properly to control AIDS, principal requirements are proposed and clinical examples are recommended as follows.

I. Principal Requirements in the Prophylaxis and Treatment of AIDS with TCM

As everyone knows, the management of AIDS with TCM is still in an exploratory stage. It is believed that through precise Evidence (or Syndrome) Differentiation and Therapy Selection, intrinsic or extrinsic conditions which influence the development of AIDS may be changed. Thus, not only symptoms may be alleviated, but the progress of disease condition may also be checked, due to the blockage of the multiplication of HIV and the elimination of its toxicity.

I) Mastery of the methodology of Evidence Differentiation, flexible application of the principles of "Treating the Same Disease with Difierent Methods" and "Treating Different Diseases with the Same Method"

Traditional Chinese doctors attach much importance to the concept of holism and the methodology of selecting therapy in accordance with Evidence Differentiation.

Every kind of disease is inseparable from its cause, its pathologic location, its pathologic nature, and its manifestations which represent the wrestling state of Healthy Energy and Pathogenic Evil. A correct Evidence Differentiation comes out from the analysis of symptoms and signs including those of the tongue, the pulse, and data of laboratory examinations. But symptoms and signs vary with the lapse of time or the different stages of disease. Hence, it is quite evident that the result of Evidence Differentiation varies with the development of the same disease. Only by careful analysis of symptoms and signs manifested at the time of treating the patient, can we obtain a judgement conforming with the actual situation.

From the infection of HIV to the development of AIDS, there is a long period of time, in which various symptoms and signs may be observed. Since its clinical manifestations differ in thousands of ways, the principle of "Treating the Same Disease with Different Methods" should be incarnated. On the other hand, since clinical manifestations caused by HIV infection are similar to those caused by other pathogenic factors, according to theories of TCM, therapeutic measures for treating other diseases may be utilized to treat HIV infection. This is the so-called principle of "Treating Different Diseases with the Same Method".

All basic principles of TCM should be observed in the prophylaxis and treatment of AIDS.

II) Exact identification of the cause and pathology of AIDS and elaborate selection of Chinese medicinal herbs to compose an effective prescription

In the management of AIDS, drugs or prescriptions selected should conform to the result of Evidence Differentiation as we have already discussed. Moreover, drugs or prescriptions which may kill HIV, protect immunologic function from being harmed, guard against opportunistic infections and other complications, and benefit the control of disease condition should be taken into consideration and adopted as far as possible. Evidently, the most important aim among these intentions is to exterminate HIV. Unfortunately up to now, special remedy for killing HIV had not been available. Under such circumstances, we lay hope on TCM, because it may alleviate symptoms, prolong survival time, and reduce death rate, even though its underlying therapeutic mechanisms remain to be explored.

HIV belongs to slow virus of the reverse transcriptive type; reverse transcriptase is needed in its replication. Its genoma assumes a form of provirus and lives in the host cell, causing latent infection. Its expression is mediated by the polymerase II of cellular RNA. After HIV has invaded human body, it encroaches lymph tissue and lymphocyte of the immune system firstly, resulting in pathologic changes of their functions. Consequently, in composing anti-HIV prescriptions, not only drugs inhibiting reverse transcriptase and cellular RNA polymerase should be selected, but those which guard lymph tissue and lymphocyte directively against encroachment must be included, thereby to block the multiple replication of HIV and the progressive deterioration of immunologic function, and to recover the immunologic function.

T peptide of 8 amino acids on protein of HIV capsule is chemotactic to mononuclear macrophage. Hence, mononuclear macrophage in human body is invaded at first and become the main host of HIV, where HIV lives in and keeps in storage. The development and maturation of these infected mononuclear macrophages are impeded, their ability of inactivating pathogens declines, leading to nonspecific immunologic deficiency, which turns into the main cause of opportunistic infection. Therefore, in composing anti-HIV prescriptions, pharmacologic action should be pointed directively towards the blockage of the multiplication of HIV in mononuclear macrophage and its proliferation, the reinforcement of the ability of mononuclear macrophage to inactivate pathogens, so as to decrease the incidence of opportunistic infection.

Furthermore, HIV invades nervous tissue at the same time, leading to disturbances of the central and the peripheral nervous system, such as progressive dementia, subacute cephalitis, peripheral neurosis, etc. Accordingly, in composing anti-HIV prescriptions, drugs which may penetrate blood brain barrier should be selected.

The above-mentioned analyses indicate that in the prophylaxis and treatment of AIDS with TCM, the premise and the crux are correct Evidence Differentiation and Therapy Selection. Through the application of TCM theories and the administration of Chinese medicinal herbs, specific remedies may be unearthed.

II. Preliminary Reports on Treating AIDS with TCM

The first report on treating AIDS with TCM in China appeared at February 1988 (Yu Juan: *Clinical Course of a White American Sufferjng from AIDS and Treated with TCM*). Thereafter, in October 1988, Wang Xuao, et al. narrated the therapeutic effect of No. 1 Prescription for AIDS in treating 3 hemophiliacs infected by HIV. From February to March in 1990, Su Chenglian reported successively his clinical experiences in treating 30 AIDS patients in Africa. In March 1991, Huang Bingshan (Heilongjiang College of TCM) and his American cooperators announced that they had treated 181 AIDS patients with Chinese medicinal herbs and acupuncture-moxibustion. These proved that TCM is both feasible and effective, and its application is in a course of spreading out.

Huang Bingshan had divided 19 cases out of 181 into three classes: bodily Asthenia accompanied with exopathy, chronic consumption, and complicated AIDS. In treating these patients, he payed close attention to essential points of raising immunocompetence, guarding against opportunistic infection, and resisting tumorigenesis, etc. Clinical symptoms of all these 19 patients were alleviated. For instance, a white, male American, 40 years of age, had been diagnosed definitely as suffering from AIDS and complicated by pulmonary infection. After 15 dosages of Chinese decoction had been taken, high fever, aversion to cold, chest pain, cough, and so forth disappeared; pressing breath was relieved apparently. 40 more dosages were administered with remarkable improvement of appetite and physical strength. 4 months later, follow-up survey proved that his disease condition was steady.

The rest 162 patients were treated with acupuncture and moxibustion. Their main symptoms alleviated significantly, the rate of symptom allevaition was 75.5%. Besides, immunologic function was improved in 139 patients. For example, a patient was diagnosed definitely as suffering from ARC. After acupuncture and moxibustion, tumescent lymph nodes shrank, all symptoms and signs disappeared, such as fever, cough, feeling of oppression in the chest, shortness of breath, diarrhea, feebleness, etc. He resumed his original work.

In order to help beginners in practising TCM, we made extracts from typical case reports cited in above-mentioned treatises and compiled them as follows:

I) Patients infected by HIV

A comparatively long latent period elapses from the invasion of HIV to the appearance of various symptoms and signs. During this period, the patient infected may remain as an asymptomatic HIV carrier, or bear manifestations of acute HIV infection. Therefore, the treatment of HIV carrier is very important to the postpone or blockage of the development of pathologic damages.

Zhejiang Research Group for Treating AIDS by Combining Traditional Chinese and Western Medicine had treated hemophiliacs infected by HIV through infusion of concentrated Factor VIII and Factor IX, as well as patients infected by HIV through other routes. **No. 1 Prescription for AIDS** and **No.2 Prescription for AIDS** were elaborated and administered to 3 and 5 cases respectively with good therapeutic results.

1. Evidence Differentiation of 3 cases infected by HIV and their treatment with **No.1 Prescription for AIDS**

From September to December in 1985, we examined blood sera of hemophiliacs who had received concentrated Factor VIII and Factor IX. These were obtained from an American pharmaceutical corporation during March 1983-June 1984. HIV antibody was ascertained by ELISA in 4 patients. All these 4 patients had received concentrated Factor VIII of the same batch number, and positive reactions were detected in both immunofluorescence assay and Western Blot test. Thus, HIV infection was definitely diagnosed. One of them died at February 1987. Through autopsy, pathologic diagnoses were established: 1) ARC; 2) hemophilic intracranial hemorrhage.

Since April 1987, we have carried out clinical and laboratory studies on the rest 3 patients systematically. Theories of TCM and techniques of modern Western Medicine were applied in their comprehensive examination. On the basis of careful Evidence typing, corresponding therapeutic principles and measures were adopted, and they were treated with prescriptions composed of Chinese medicinal herbs.

These 3 male patients were at the age of 9, 16, and 28. Their common symptoms and signs were as follows: recurrent spontaneous escape of blood within joints, pale or slightly pale complexion, extreme fatigability, perspiration, obvious emaciation, poor appetite. Nevertheless, their urination, defecation, and daily lives were normal. In 1 case, the tongue was pale; in the other 2 cases, tongues were reddened with white and thin coating. Their pulse conditions were thready and rapid.

Results of laboratory examination: slight or moderate decrease of hemoglobin; slight decrease in counts of WBC, thrombocyte, and lymphocyte in 2 patients; remarkable decrease of OKT_4 (29.5%, 28.0%, and 31.5% respectively) and remarkable increase of T_8 (49.0%, 54.0%, and 43.0% respectively); the ratio of T_4/T_8) was significantly lower than normal standard (0.60, 0.52, and 0.74 respectively); negative OT (1:2000) skin test in all 3 patients.

Histories of recurrent spontaneous escape of blood within joints suggested that there were intrinsic factors of protracted Asthenia of Healthy Energy. Under such circumstances, HIV infection further impaired Healthy Energy. Consequently, there were manifestations of Qi Asthenia, such as weariness, perspiration, pale complexion, emaciation, etc. Functional defect of T lymphocyte was also confirmed by laboratory examination.

According to findings of current research into the combination of TCM and Western Medicine, hypofunction of cellular immunity is one of the characteristics of Qi Asthenia of Solid and Hollow Organs. Therefore, the feature in common of these 3 patients was Qi Asthenia. On the other hand, in view of the fact that reddened tongue was observed in 2 of them and thready, rapid pulse was observed in all of them, there was Yin Asthenia at the same time. Hence the conclusion of Evidence Differentiation was deficiency of both Qi and Yin in this group of patients.

It is clear that priority should be given to the support of Healthy Energy. Accordingly, Chinese medicinal herbs which may replenish the deficiency of both Qi and Yin, safeguard the cellular immunologic function, and strengthen the body resistance must be selected and a prescription was elaborated. It was named **No.1 Prescription for AIDS**. Later, its name was changed into **No.1 Chinese Prescription**.

After these patients had been treated with this prescription for nearly one year, their general conditions were improved apparently. Frequency of recurrent spontaneous escape of blood within joints was reduced, bodily strength was invigorated. The growth and development of 2 adolescent patients became normal. Most manifestations of the deficiency of both Qi and Yin were alleviated.

Results of laboratory examination: normal range of RBC, WBC, and lymphocytes in peripheral blood; increase of OKT_4, decrease of T_8, elevation of the ratio of T_4/T_8. These data approaches their normal criteria at the end of the therapeutic course, indicating that **No.1 Chinese Prescription** was effective in reinforcing physical strength, replenishing the body, and protecting cellular immunity against damage. So far, no adverse or toxic reaction occurred. This prescription has been considered as one of the effective remedies in treating HIV infection by specialists in this domain. Further researches are in progress.

2. Evidence Differentiation and treatment of 5 cases infected by HIV with **No. 2 Prescription for AIDS**

This group includes 3 hemophiliacs mentioned above. Their disease conditions were steady and had been followed up for more than one year. The other 2 cases were male patients infected by HIV while working abroad, and were 22 and 42 years of age. At April and May in 1990, their blood sera were examined by ELISA, IFA, and Western Blot test. All results were positive. HIV infection was definitely diagnosed.

Findings at the first visit: recurrent hemarthrosis in 3 cases; fatigability after physical activities in 5 cases; body weight less than normal standard but with normal appetite, urination, and defectation in 2 cases; slightly pale complexion in 3 cases, ruddy complexion in 2 cases; pale tongue in 2 cases, reddened tongue in 2 cases, pale reddened tongue in 1 case; white and thin lingual coating in 3 cases, greasy and thin lingual coating in 2 cases; pulse conditions of all these patients were thready and rapid. Results of laboratory examination: quantity of hemoglobin, count and classification of WBC, and counts of lymphocytes and thrombocytes were within normal standard in the main. Detection of subgroups of T lymphocytes: ratio of T_4/T_8 remained within 1.0-1.30 in 3 cases, and at 0.54 and 0.43 respectively in the other 2 cases.

3 cases had been infected by HIV for 6-7 years; in the other

2 cases, positive HIV antibody had been detected for more than 1 year. It goes without saying that Healthy Energy was depleted gradually due to the protracted lingering of Pathogenic Evil. Loss of body weight, fatigability, pictures of the tongue, and conditions of the pulse all suggested the Asthenia of Both Qi and Yin.

In line with the above-mentioned analyses, therapeuitc principle of Supporting Healthy Energy to Eliminate Pathogenic Evil was adopted. Seven Chinese medicinal herbs which may replenish Asthenia of both Qi and Yin, protect cellular immunity against HIV, and regulate the function of humoral immunity were selected to compose a new prescription, **No. 2 Prescription for AIDS**. After its decoction had been administered for more than 10 months, physical strength of these patients was invigorated and they began to continue their normal study, work, or daily life. Detection of subgroups of T lymphocytes had been carried out in 4 patients, the ratio of OKT_4/OKT_8 was over 1.0 generally.

These results indicated that **No. 2 Prescription for AIDS** was effective in ameliorating clinical symptoms, safeguarding immunologic function, and preventing the patient from secondary infection. Further observations and researches are in progress.

II) Evidence Differentiation and treatment of ARC and AIDS

ARC and AIDS result from serious damage of immunologic function caused by the multitudinous replication and proliferation of HIV. Such patients had been observed and treated abroad by our medical scholars in recent years.

Fever, cough, diarrhea, emaciation, feebleness, and so forth occur in most of these patients and may be treated by therapeutic measures recorded in TCM books, such as those of consumptive disease caused by internal damage, Defence-Energy-Nutrient-Blood Systems in epidemic febrile disease, and Three Yin Syndromes in exogenous febrile disease. Specifically, since there are various types and degrees of fever and hemorrhage to a certain extent from beginning to end, they may be treated with principles of epidemic febrile disease in its early and intermediate stage, and those of consumptive disease in advanced stage. Certainly, such principles should be handled flexibly in accordance with individual conditions.

Detailed reports on treating AIDS with TCM are rare. In order to explain the methodology of Evidence Differentiation and Therapy Selection in treating AIDS, case reports written by Yu Juan and Su Cheng Lian are cited as follows:

1. Case report from Yu Juan

A white, male American, 39 years of age, seeked medical advice because of systemic lymphadenectasis for 3-4 years; and fatigability, anorexia, chronic diarrhea for more than 8 months. So far he had not received any systematic treatment.

The diarrhea was watery and took place 3-4 times daily. It was mixed with food dregs but without pus or blood. Its smell was sour and foul. No abnormal findings were detected by routine stool examination. The patient could not persevere with daily work due to somasthenia. There were frequent catching cold, sustained feeling of swelling throat, subjective fever (normal body temperature), thirst, dry mouth, depressive mood, self-depreciation, malancholy, or even intention to commit suicide. During a long period of more than 10 years before he came to clinic, his sexual behaviour was frequent, perverted and out of control. He indulged himself in homosexuality with more than 20 young males around 25-26 years of age. These sexual partners suffered from fatigability, feebleness, lymphadenectasis, chronic diarrhea, etc. and died successively four years ago. Two years ago, he received HIV antibody examination. The result was positive twice. AIDS was definitely diagnosed.

Physical examination: weariness, emaciation, sallow complexion, knitting of eyebrows, obvious congestion of the throat, slight enlargement of the tonsil; general lymphadenectasis (about 3×4×2 cm) in submaxillary, post-sternocleidomastoid, subaxillary, and inguinal regions, these lymph nodes were movable and without tenderness; liver edge, 2 cm below the costal margin; spleen, palpable; examination of the heart and the lung, negative; NS examination, no pathologic reflex. Reddened and tender tongue with longitudinal fissures; reddened and prickly margin of the lingual tip; yellow, greasy, and thin coating of the tongue, yellow and thick coating at the lingual root. Candida culture of exfoliative epithelia from the lingual tip, positive. Pulse rate, over 90/min. Pulse condition, bow-string and slippery.

Laboratory examination: HIV antibody, positive; routine examination of peripheral blood, normal; albumin, 42g/L; globulin, 28g/L; A/G = 1.5; SGOT, 136 IU/L (normal, 0-41 IU/L); SGPT, 268 IU/L (normal, 0-45IU/L); prothrombin time, 15.2 sec (normal, 11-13 sec); prothrombin activity, 43% (normal, 70-100%). The rest 22 items of blood biochemical examination, normal.

Evidence Differentiation: Chronic Spleen Asthenia, soakage of Wetness, invasion of Heat Toxin, accumulation and fermentation of Turbidity, Wetness, Heat, and Toxin; Qi and Blood Systems are involved. In short, it is a Syndrome of Heat Toxin.

According to theories of TCM, the Root of his disease is Yang Asthenia of Spleen and Kidney, the Branch is Sthenia. Therefore, it should be treated with "clear away Heat, resolve Toxin, eliminate Wetness, and cool Blood" firstly. After that,

Kidney should be benefited, Spleen strengthened, and Heart nourished.

At the initial stage, Sweet Dew Detoxication Pill ("Compendium on Epidemic Febrile Diseases" by Wang Mengying) was adopted as a principal prescription, modified in compliance with the disease condition. Chinese medicinal herbs which may clear away Heat, resolve Toxin, and cool Blood were administered early or late, such as Herba Scutellariae Barbatae, Herba Oldenlandiae Diffusae, Flos Lonicerae, Fructus Forsythiae, Folium Isatidis, Radix Isatidis, Cortex Moutan Radicis, Fructus Gardeniae, etc. In addition, adjuvant drugs such as Fructus Hordei Germinatus, Fructus Crataegi, etc. , which may remove stagnation and promote digestion were added.

After such prescription had been taken continuously for 4 months, his symptoms were alleviated, vitality and physical strength were improved, loose stool turned into formed or soft faeces, his appetite was recovered and ordinary diets could be taken. The patient began to go in for a half-day work. His tongue changed from reddened colour to pale red, but was still enlarged, moistened, teeth-printed, and fissured; its coating was white and thin. The pulse condition was bow-string like and slippery, the rapid pulse disappeared (64-72/min). SGOT descended to 91 IU/L, SGPT descended to 182 IU/L. Although no significant change was observed in general physical signs, the patient was full of confidence in taking Traditional Chinese decoctions.

In view of the fact that the Pathogenic Evil, Heat Toxin, had been frustrated, manifestations of Wetness and Turbidity had been mitigated, only deficiency of both Qi and Yin was still apparent, the principal prescription was changed from Sweet Dew Detoxication Pill to Powder for Restoring Pulse Beat in the second stage. The latter may invigorate Primordial Qi and nourish Yin. Adjuvant drugs which may nourish Yin and promote the production of body fluid were also selected, such as Radix Scrophulariae, Radix Rehmanniae, Fructus Ligustri Lucidi, Herba Ecliptae, etc.

Physical strength of the patient was restored gradually. He had a good appetite and his diarrhea disappeared. After 9 months, results of laboratory examination were as follows: SGOT, 73IU/L; SGPT, 169IU/L; albumin, 45g/L, globulin, 25g/L, A/G = 1.8. But the disease condition was not steady. Two months later, herpes zoster occurred on the right side of his loin (T12-L1). There were pain, fever, and a large number of blisters. Chinese medicinal herbs which may clear away Heat and cool Blood were administered, such as Rhizoma Coptidis, Folium Isatidis, Radix Arnebiae seu Lithospermi, Cortex Moutan Radicis, etc. Two weeks later, skin lesions became scabbed and extinct, the pain faded away. Thereafter, sporadic, pinpoint red spots appeared twice on the medial side of the patient's forearm. At that time, the fragility test of blood vessels was positive. By modifying the remedy to suit the case, they disappeared quickly and then no relapse occurred.

After such treatment had been carried out for 1 year, his appetite and defecation became normal, his vitality took a turn for the better, and his lymph nodes shrank obviously. He could persevere in a fulltime study. Results of return visit examination were as follows: pale, moist, and enlarged tongue proper; deep, thready, and slippery pulse; palpitation, blurred vision, dizziness, etc. A prescription for supporting Healthy Energy, Decoction for Invigorating Spleen and Nourishing Heart, was selected, putting Radix Astragali seu Hedysari in an important position. Two weeks later, the palpitation was alleviated; the patient could sleep soundly and entreated us to continue such treatment.

Consequently, supporting Healthy Energy with Decoction

for Invigorating Spleen and Nourishing Heart was the principal therapeutic measure in the third stage. Adjuvant drugs were Semen Cuscutae, Herba Epimedii, Fructus Ligustri Lucidi, etc., which may invigorate Kidney Yang and nourishing Kidney Yin were administered alternately, and to benefit Heart and Spleen at the same time, as well as to improve the humoral and cellular immunologic function.

From May 1986 to September 1987, the above-mentioned treatment had been carried out. The disease condition remained steady. The patient said he had not catch cold for several months, and no sore throat occurred; both appetite and physical strength were good. The count of T helper lymphocyte was 91/mm .

In December 1987, the patient was followed up. His disease condition was steady.

2. Case report from Su Chenglian

The patient was a male, married soldier, aged 33. He seeked medical advice because of diarrhea, emaciation, feebleness, and recurrent fever for more than 1 year, which had been aggravated for 2 months.

About 1 year ago, the following symptoms and signs appeared: watery diarrhea, abdominal distension and pain, aching of limbs, feebleness, gradual emaciation, frequent fever, aversion to cold, dizziness, palpitation, cough with a small amount of phlegm, feeling of oppression in the chest, anorexia, nausea, unsound sleep, etc.

At the time of seeking medical advice, his diarrhea took place 7-10 times daily; HIV test, positive. AIDS was diagnosed definitely. From June 27, 1988, the patient began to receive TCM treatment.

Physical examination: temperature, 37.2°C; pulse rate, 120/min.; lymphadenectasis (about 0.5 × 0.6 cm) on both sides of the neck; liver edge was palpated 1.5 cm below the costal margin, it was soft and without tenderness. The spleen could not be palpated. Body weight, 40 kg. Reddened tongue with petechiae on both sides, yellow and thin lingual coating. Pulse condition, thready and rapid.

Laboratory examination: hemoglobin, 131g/L; WBC, 8.0×10^9/L; neutrophil, 50%; lymphocyte, 38%; mononuclear leukocyte, 6%; eosinophil, 6%; blood platelet, normal.

Evidence Differentiation: Deficiency of Healthy Energy, Asthenia and impairment of Spleen-Stomach, internal accumulation of Evil Toxin.

Therapeutic principle: Supporting Healthy Energy, eliminating Evil Toxin, cultivating and invigorating Spleen-Stomach.

Recipe: Mixture for Supporting Healthy Energy, combined with Decoction for Invigorating Middle Energizer and Benefiting Qi, and modified Minor Decoction of Bupleurum. Moreover, adjuvant drugs such as Rhizoma Smilacis Glabrae, Radix Isatidis, etc. were selected.

After 10 dosages had been taken, cough and shortness of breath were somewhat alleviated, but other symptoms remained the same. Diarrhea took place more than 10 times daily; reddened tongue with yellow and thin coating; thready and rapid pulse. Accordingly, Radix Isatidis and Radix Scutellariae were removed from the original prescription, baked ginger, Fructus Chebulae, and roasted Radix Aucklandiae were added.

After 6 dosages had been taken, the frequency of diarrhea decreased to 3-4 times daily. The other symptoms were also alleviated. Over 20 dosages of this prescription were taken successively, then his diarrhea was controlled. Formed stool was defecated once or twice daily.

But not long after that, his diarrhea relapsed. Morning diarrhea occurred for 3-4 times daily; dull abdominal pain, feebleness, aversion to cold, cold limbs; white and thin coating of the tongue; deep and thready pulse. These indicated Yang Asthenia of Spleen-Kidney or "Fire fails to generate Earth".

Therapeutic principle: Warming and invigorating Spleen-Kidney, stopping diarrhea with astringents.

Recipe: Mixture for Supporting Healthy Energy, combined with modified Pill of Four Miraculous Drugs; and Pill for Invigorating Kidney Energy (from *Synopsis of the Golden Chamber*) concurrently.

After 14 dosages had been taken, the diarrhea was controlled in the main. Formed stool was defected 1-2 times daily. Most symptoms and signs such as dizziness, palpitation, cough, anorexia, nausea, aversion to cold, cold limbs, etc. disappeared. There were only feebleness, slight yellow and thin coating of the tongue, and thready pulse. Hemoglobin, 112g/L; total count and classification of WBC, normal; body weight, 39 kg.

On September 29, 1988, the patient was discharged from the hospital at his request.

APPENDIX Prescriptions Cited in This Book

1. Decoction Consisting of Eight Precious Ingredients

Radix Angelicae Sinensis, Rhizoma Ligustici Chuanxiong, Radix Paeoniae Alba, Rhizoma Rehmanniae Praeparatae, Radix Ginseng, Rhizoma Atractylodis Macrocephalae, Poria coccos, Radix Glycyrrhizae.

2. Two Solstices Pill

Herba Ecliptae, Fructus Ligustri Lucidi.

3. Decoction of Radix Asparagi, Radix Ophiopogonis, Rhizoma Anemarrhenae, and Bulus Fritillariae

Radix Asparagi, Radix Ophiopogonis, Rhizoma Anemarrhenae, Bulbus Fritillariae.

4. Bolus for Eight-Immortals' Longevity

Rhizoma Rehmanniae Praeparatae, Fructus Corni, Rhizoma Dioscoreae, Poria coccos, Rhizoma Alismatis, Cortex Moutan Radicis, Radix Ophiopogonis, Fructus Schisandrae.

5. Seven Blessings' Drink

Radix Ginseng, Rhizoma Rehmanniae Praeparatae, Radix Angelicae Sinensis, Rhizoma Atractylodis Macrocephalae, Radix Glycyrrhizae, Semen Ziziphi Spinosae, Radix Polygalae.

6. Decoction (Bolus) of Ten Powerful Tonics

Radix Ginseng, Rhizoma Angelicae Sinensis, Radix Astragali seu Hedysari, Radix Rehmanniae Praeparatae, Poria coccos, Radix Paeoniae Alba, Rhizoma Atractylodis Macrocephalae, Rhizoma Ligustici Chuanxiong, Radix Glycyrrhizae, Cortex

Cinnamomi.

7. Radix Ginseng Pill for Nourishing Nutrient System

Radix Ginseng, Cortex Cinnamomi, Fructus Schisandrae, Radix Paeoniae Alba, Radix Astragali seu Hedysari, Rhizoma Atractylodis Macrocephalae, Poria coccos, Radix Angelicae Sinensis, Rhizoma Rehmanniae Praeparatae, Pericarpium Citri Reticulatae, Radix Glycyrrhizae, Radix Polygalae.

8. Bolus for Replenishing Yin Greatly

Cortex Phellodendri, Rhizoma Anemarrhenae, Rhizoma Rehmanniae Praeparatae, Plastrum Testudinis, Spinal marrow of pig.

9. Decoction for Replenishing Primordial Essence Greatly

Radix Ginseng, Rhizoma Dioscoreae, Rhizoma Rehmanniae Praeparatae, Cortex Eucommiae, Radix Angelicae Sinensis, Fructus Corni, Fructus Lycii, Radix Glycyrrhizae.

10. Big Pearl for Wind Syndrome

Radix Paeoniae Alba, Colla Corii Asini, Plastrum Testudinis, Radix Rehmanniae, Fructus Cannabis, Fructus Shisandrae, Concha Ostreae, Radix Ophiopogonis, Radix Glycyrrhizae praeparata, Fresh yolk, Carapax Trionycis.

11. Minor Golden Pellet

Resina Liquidambaris, Radix Aconiti Kusnezoffii, Faeces Trogopterorum, Lumbricus, Semen Momordicae, Resina Commiphorae Myrrhae, Resina Olibani, Radix Angelicae Sinensis, Moschus, Carbon of Chinese ink.

12. Minor Decoction of Radix Bupleuri

Radix Bupleuri, Radix Scutellariae, Rhizoma Pinelliae, Radix Ginseng, Radix Glycyrrhizae Praeparata, Rhizoma Zingiberis Recens, Fructus Ziziphi Jujubae.

13. Bolus of Six Drugs Including Radix Rehmanniae

Rhizoma Rehmanniae Praeparatae, Fructus Corni, Poria coccos, Rhizoma Alismatis, Rhizoma Dioscoreae, Cortex Moutan

Radicis.

14. Pill of Six Miraculous Drugs

Western Calculus Bovis, Borneolum, Margarita, Venenum Bufonis, Realgar, Moschus.

15. Wen's Experiential Prescription

Radix Polygoni Multiflori, Bombyx Batryticatus, Periostracum Cicadae, Flos Lonicerae, Fructus Kochiae, Cortex Dictamni Radicis, Corium Erinacei, Cortex Phellodendri, Rhizoma Atractylodis, Radix Gentianae, Cortex Moutan Radicis, Rhizoma Smilacis Glabrae, Herba Artemisiae Scopariae, Excrementum Bombycis.

16. (Experiential) Prescription for Relieving Itching and Calming Wind

Radix Rehmanniae, Cortex Moutan Radicis, Radix Paeoniae Rubra, Radix Salviae Miltiorrhizae, Os Draconis, Concha Ostreae, Fructus Tribuli, Radix Scrophulariae, Radix Glycyrrhizae, Cortex Dictamni Radicis.

17. Bolus for Resolving Scrofula Interiorly

Spica Prunellae, Sargassum, Radix Trichosanthis, Bulbus Fritillariae Thunbergii, Sea Clam-shell. Fructus Aurantii, Fructus Forsythiae, Radix Ampelopsis, Nitrum, Halitum, Radix Angleicae Sinensis, Radix Rehmanniae, Rhizoma Rehmanniae Praeparatae, Radix Scrophulariae, Radix Platycodi, Herba Menthae, Radix Glycyrrhizae.

18. Decoction of Five Roots

Rhizoma Imperatae, Radix Isatidis, Radix Trichosanthis, Radix Sanguisorbae, Radix Arnebiae seu Lithospermi, Cortex Moutan Radicis.

19. Decoction of Four Noble Drugs

Radix Ginseng, Rhizoma Atractylodis Macrocephalae, Poria coccos, Radix Glycyrrhizae Praeparata.

20. Decoction of Four Drugs

Radix Angelicae Sinensis, Rhizoma Rehmanniae Praeparatae, Radix Paeoniae Alba, Rhizoma Liguistici Chuanxiong.

21. Pill of Four Miraculous Drugs

Fructus Psoraleae, Fructus Schisandrae, Semen Myristicae, Fructus Euodiae, Rhizoma Zingiberis Recens, Fructus Ziziphi Jujubae.

22. White Tiger Decoction

Gypsum Fibrosum, Rhizoma Anemarrhenae, Radix Glycyrrhizae Praeparata, Semen Oryzae Sativae.

23. Radix Pulsatillae Decoction

Radix Pulsatillae, Rhizoma Coptidis, Cortex Phellodendri, Cortex Fraxini.

24. Pill of Alumen and Radix Curcumae

Alumen, Radix Curcumae.

25. Decoction for Invigorating Spleen and Nourishing Heart

Rhizoma Atractylodis Macrocephalae, Poria coccos, Radix Astragali seu Hedysari, Arillus Longan, Semen Ziziphi Spinosae, Radix Ginseng, Radix Aucklandiae, Radix Glycyrrhizae Praeparata, Radix Angelicae Sinensis, Radix Polygalae, Rhizoma Zingiberis Recens, Fructus Ziziphi Jujubae.

26. Sweet Dew Pellet (Powder) for Detoxification

Talcum, Herba Artemisiae Scopariae, Radix Scutellariae, Rhizoma Acori Graminei, Caulis Akebiae, Bulbus Fritillariae Cirrhosae, Rhizoma Belamcandae, Fructus Forsythiae, Herba Menthae, Semen Amomi Cardamomi, Herba Agastachis.

27. Decoction of Radix Gentianae for Purging Liver Fire

Radix Gentianae, Radix Scutellariae, Fructus Gardeniae, Rhizoma Alismatis, Caluis Akebiae, Semen Plantaginis, Radix Angelicae Sinensis, Radix Bupleuri, Radix Rehmanniae, Radix Glycyrrhizae.

28. Bolus for Restoring the Left Kidney

Rhizoma Rehmanniae Praeparatae, Rhizoma Dioscoreae,

Fructus Corni, Fructus Lycii, Semen Cuscutae, Radix Achyranthis Bidentatae, Colla Cornus Cervi, Colla Plastri Testudinis.

29. Jade Screen Powder

Radix Astragali seu Hedysari, Rhizoma Atractylodis Macrocephalae, Radix Ledebouriellae.

30. Powder for Restoring Pulse Beat

Radix Ginseng, Radix Ophiopogonis, Fructus Schisandrae.

31. Decoction of Radix Angeicae Sinensis for Replenishing Blood

Radix Angelicae Sinensis, Radix Astragali seu Hedysari.

32. Bezoar Bolus (Powder) for Resurrection (Coated with gold foil)

Calculus Bovis, Radix Curcumae, Cornu Rhinoceri, Radix Scutellariae, Rhizoma Coptidis, Realgar, Fructus Gardeniae, Cinnabaris, Borneolum, Moschus, Margarita.

33. Treasured Bolus

Radix Rehmanniae, Cornu Rhinoceri, Carapax Eretmochelydis. Succinum, Cinnabaris, Realgar, Resina dryobalanops Aromticae, Moschus, Calculus Bovis, Benzoinum, Gold foil, Silver foil.

34. Radix Rehmanniae Decoction

Radix Rehmanniae, Radix Morindae Officinalis, Fructus Corni, Herba Dendrobii, Herba Cistanchis, Radix Aconiti Praeparata, Fructus Schisandrae, Cortex Cinnamomi, Poria coccos, Radix Ophiopogonis, Rhizoma Acori Graminei, Radix Polygalae, Herba Menthae, Rhizoma Zingiberis Recens, Fructus Ziziphi Jujubae.

35. Bolus for Rehabilitation

Agkistrodon, Radix Ginseng, Radix Clematidis, Radix Notoginseng, Lignum Aquilariae Resinatum, Rhizoma Gastrodiae, Calculus Bovis, Cinnabaris.

36. Decoction (Bolus) for Invigorating Middle Energizer and

Benefiting Qi

Radix Astragali seu Hedysari, Rhizoma Atractylodis Macrocephalae, Pericarpium Citri Reticulata, Rhizoma Cimicifugae, Radix Bupleuri, Radix Angelicae Sinensis. Radix Ginseng, Radix Glycyrrhizae Praeparata.

37. Decoction of Radix Adenophorae Strictae and Radix Ophiopogonis

Radix Adenophorae Strictae, Radix Ophiopogonis, Rhizoma Polygonati Odorati, Radix Glycyrrhizae, Folium Mori, Semen Dolichoris Alba, Radix Trichosanthis.

38. Bolus of Fructus Lycii-Flos Chrysanthemi and Rhizoma Rehmanniae Praeparatae.

Fructus Lycii, Flos Chrysanthemi, Cortex Moutan Radicis, Fructus Corni, Rhizoma Dioscoreae, Rhizoma Alismatis, Poria coccos, Rhizoma Rehmanniae Praeparatae.

39. Bolus for Treating Epilepsy

Rhizoma Typhonii, Rhizoma Arisaematis, Rhizoma Pinelliae Praeparata, Fructus Gleditsiae Abnormalis, Bombyx Batryticatus, Zaocys, Scolopendra, Scorpio, Alumen, Realgar, Cinnabaris.

40. Placenta Hominis Bolus for Energetic Rehabilitation

Placenta Hominis, Rhizoma Rehmanniae Praeparatae, Radix Asparagi, Radix Ophiopogonis, Plastrum Testudinis, Cortex Phellodendri, Cortex Eucommiae, Radix Achyranthis Bidentatae.

41. Powder (Bolus) of Radix Ginseng, Poria coccos, and Rhizoma Atractylodis Macrocephalae

Radix Ginseng, Poria coccos, Rhizoma Atractylodis Macrocephalae, Semen Dolichoris Album, Rhizoma Dioscoreae, Semen Nelumbinis, Fructus Amomi, Semen Coicis, Radix Platycodi, Radix Glycyrrhizae, Pericarpium Citri Reticulatae.

42. Pill for Calming Epilepsy

Rhizoma Gastrodiae, Bulbus Fritillariae Cirrhosae, Arisaema cum Bile, Rhizoma Pinelliae, Poria coccos, Poria cum Ligno Hospite, Radix Salviae Miltiorrhizae, Radix Ophiopogonis, Scorpio, Bombyx Batryticatus, Succinum, Cinnabaris, Succus Bombosae, Juice of Rhizoma Zingiberis Recens, Radix Glycyrrhizae.

43. Golden Lock Pill for Consolidating Kidney Essence

Semen Astragali Complanati, Fructus Tribuli, Semen Euryales, Stamen Nelumbinis, Os Draconis, Concha Ostreae,(Semen Nelumbinis).

44. Prescription for Nourishing Blood to Stop Wind

Radix Astragali seu Hedysari, Radix Angelicae Sinensis, Radix Paeoniae Alba, Rhizoma Ligustici Chuanxiong, Flos Carthami, Radix Scrophulariae, Herba Schizonepetae, Fructus Tribuli, Radix Glycyrrhizae.

45. Powder of Radix Rubiae

Radix Rubiae, Cacumen Biotae, Radix Scutellariae, Radix Rehmanniae, Colla Corii Asini, Radix Glycyrrhizae.

46. Pellet of Miraculous Rhinoceros Horn

Cornu Rhinoceri, Rhizoma Acori Graminei, Radix Scutellariae, Radix Rehmanniae, Flos Lonicerae, Faeces water, Fructus Forsythiae, Radix Arnebiae seu Lithospermi, Radix Isatidis, Semen Sojae Praeparatum, Radix Scrophulariae, Radix Trichosanthis.

47. Decoction for Eliminating Phlegm

Rhizoma Pinelliae Praeparatae, Rhizoma Arisaematis Praeparatae, Poria coccos, Fructus Aurantii Immaturus, Pericarpium Citri Reticulatae, Radix Ginseng, Rhizoma Acori Graminei, Caulis Bambusae in Taeniam, Radix Glycyrrhizae, Rhizoma Zingiberis Recens.

48. Decoction of Four Drugs with Semen Persicae and Flos Carthami

Semen Persicae, Flos Carthami, Radix Angelicae Sinensis, Rhizoma Ligustici Chuanxiong, Radix Paeoniae, Radix Rehmanniae.

49. Pill for Resolving Scrofula

Radix Scrophulariae, Concha Ostreae Usta, Bulbus Fritillariae Thunbergii.

50. Radix Bupleuri Powder for Dispersing Liver Qi

Radix Bupleuri, Pericarpium Citri Reticulatae, Radix Paeoniae, Fructus Aurantii, Radix Glycyrrhizae Praeparata, Rhizoma Ligustici Chuanxiong, Rhizoma Cyperi.

51. Powder for Clearing Away Hectic Fever

Radix Stellariae, Rhizoma Picrorhizae, Radix Gentianae Macrophyllae, Carapax Trionycis, Cortex Lycii Radicis, Herba Artemisiae Chinghao, Rhizoma Anemarrhenae, Radix Glycyrrhizae.

52. Decoction for Clearing Away Heat in Nutrient System

Cornu Rhinoceri, Radix Salviae Miltiorrhizae, Rhizoma Coptidis, Radix Scrophulariae, Radix Rehmanniae, Radix Ophiopogonis, Flos Lonicerae, Fructus Forsythiae, Leaf buds of Herba Lophatheri.

53. Decoction for Opening Aperture and Activating Blood

Radix Paeoniae Rubra, Rhizoma Ligustici Chuanxiong, Semen Persicae, Flos Carthami, Allium Fistulosum, Rhizoma Zingiberis Recens, Fructus Ziziphi Jujubae, Moschus.

54. Pill for Clearing Away Lung Heat and Resolving Phlegm

Radix Scutellariae, Fructus Gardeniae, Radix Platycodi, Radix Ophiopogonis, Cortex Mori Radicis, Bulbus Fritillariae, Rhizoma Anemarrhenae, Semen Trichosanthis, Exocarpium Citri Grandis, Poria coccos, Radix Glycyrrhizae.

55. Pill for Clearing Away Heart Fire and Expelling Phlegm

Radix et Rhizoma Rhei, Radix Scutellariae, Lapis Chloriti, Cornu Rhinoceri, Spina Gleditsiae, Cinnabaris, Lignum Aquilariae Resinatum, Moschus.

56. Powder of Margarita and Calculus Bovis

Margarita, Calculus Bovis.

57. Bolus for Walking with Energetic Strides

Rhizoma Anemarrhenae, Cortex Phellodendri, Rhizoma Rehmanniae Praeparatae, Plastrum Testudinis, Radix Angelicae Sinensis, Radix Paeoniae Alba, Os Tigris, Radix Achyranthis Bidentatae, Herba Cynomorii, Pericarpium citri Reticulatae, Rhizoma Zingiberis, Mutton.

58. Radix Astragali seu Hedysari Drink for Restoring Pulse Beat

Radix Astragali seu Hedysari, Radix Codonopsis Pilosulae, Radix Ophiopogonis, Fructus Schisandrae.

59. Radix Astragali seu Hedysari Decoction for Invigorating Middle Energizer

Radix Astragali seu Hedysari, Ramulus Cinnamomi, Radix Glycyrrhizae Praeparata, Fructus Ziziphi Jujubae, Radix Paeoniae, Rhizoma Zingiberis Recens, Malt sugar.

60. Bolus for Regulating Middle Energizer

Radix Ginseng, Rhizoma Zingiberis, Rhizoma Atractylodis Macrocephalae, Radix Glycyrrhizae Praeparata.

61. Polyporus Umbellatus Decoction

Polyporus Umbellatus, Poria coccos, Rhizoma Alismatis, Colla Corii Asini, Talcum.

62. Decoction for Clearing Away Pestilent Evil and Detoxification

Gypsum Fibrosum, Radix Rehmanniae, Cornu Rhinoceri, Rhizoma Coptidis, Rhizoma Anemarrhenae, Radix Paeoniae Rubra, Fructus Forsythiae, Radix Scrophulariae, Radix Glycyrrhizae, Cortex Moutan Radicis, Fructus Gardeniae, Radix Platycodi, Radix Scutellariae, Herba Lophatheri.

63. Powder of Fructus Forsythiae and Flos Lonicerae

Fructus Forsythiae, Flos Lonicerae, Herba Lophatheri, Spica Schizonepetae, Fructus Arctii, Semen Sojae Praeparatum, Herba Menthae, Rhizoma Phragmitis, Radix Platycodi, Radix Glycyrrhizae.

64. Bolus for Arousing Spleen

Radix Ginseng, Rhizoma Atractylodis Macrocephalae, Poria coccos, Radix Glycyrrhizae, Pericarpium Citri Reticulatae, Rhizoma Dioscoreae, Semen Nelumbinis, Fructus Crataegi, Rhizoma Alismatis.

65. Bolus of Western Calculus Bovis

Western Calculus Bovis, Moschus, Resina Commiphorae Myrrhae, Resina Olibani.

67. Purplish Golden Lozenge

Radix Knoxiae, Bulbus Cremastrae, Semen Euphorbiae Lathyridis, Moschus, Realgar, Cinnabaris, Galla Chinensis.

69. Purplish Snow (Powder or Pellet)

Gypsum Fibrosum, Rhizoma Cimicifugae, Calcitum, Flos Syzygii Aromatici, Talcum, Natrii Sulfas, Magnetitum, Sal Nitri, Radix Scrophulariae, Cornu Rhinoceri, Radix Aucklandiae, Cornu Antelopis, Lignum Aquilariae Resinatum, Moschus, Cinnabaris, Radix Glycyrrhizae.

68. Decoction of Cornu Rhinoceri and Radix Rehmanniae

Cornu Rhinoceri, Radix Rehmanniae, Radix Paenoiae, Cortex Moutan Radicis.

69. Radix Puerariae Decoction

Radix Puerariae, Herba Ephedrae, Ramulus Cinnamomi, Radix Paeoniae, Radix Glycyrrhizae, Fructus Ziziphi Jujubae, Rhizoma Zingiberis Recens.

70. Decoction of Radix Puerariae, Radix Scutellariae, and Rhizoma Coptidis

Radix Puerariae, Radix Scutellariae, Rhizoma Coptidis, Radix Glycyrrhizae Praeparata.

71. Powder of Tin-like Ingredients

Clastic ivory, Indigo Naturalis, Uroctea (carbonized), Human Finger Nail, Margarita, Borneolum, Calculus Bovis.

72. Powder of Indigo Naturalis and Concha Meretricis seu Cyclinae

Indigo Naturalis, Concha Meretricis seu Cyclinae.

73. Pill of Venenum Bufonis

Venenum Bufonis, Realgar, Cinnabaris, Eulota Peliomphala, Calcitum, Calomelas, Aerugo, Resina Boswelliae Carterii, Resina Commiphorae Myrrhae, Moschus, Alumen Exsiccatum, Chalcanthitum.

74. Pill of Decocted Carapax Trionycis

Carapax Trionycis, Rhizoma Belamcandae, Radix Scutellariae, Radix Bupleuri, Armadillidium Vulgare, Radix et Rhizoma Rhei, Rhizoma Zingiberis, Radix Paeoniae, Ramulus Cinnamomi, Semen Lepidii seu Descurainiae, Folium Pyrrosiae, Cortex Magnoliae Officinalis, Cortex Moutan Radicis, Herba Dianthi, Flos Campsis, Rhizoma Pinelliae, Radix Ginseng, Eupolyphaga seu Steleophaga, Colla Corii Asini, Nidus Vespae, Natrii Sulfas, Roach, Semen Persicae.

75. Sweet Dew Bolus for Nourishing Yin

Radix Rehmanniae, Rhizoma Rehmanniae Praeparatae, Radix Asparagi, Radix Ophiopogonis, Radix Scrophulariae, Folium Eriobotryae, Herba Dendrobii, Herba Artemisiae Scopariae, Radix Scutellariae, Fructus Auranti, Radix Glycyrrhizae.

76. Pill or Powder for Ease and Free

Radix Bupleuri, Radix Angelicae Sinensis, Radix Paeoniae Alba, Rhizoma Atractylodis Macrocephalae, Poria coccos, Radix Glycyrrhizae Praeparata, Herba Menthae, Rhizoma Zingiberis (stewed).

77. Pill for Arousing Dissipation

Realgar, Moschus, Resina Olibani, Resina Commiphorae Myrrhae.

REFERENCES

1. Yellow Emperor: Canon of Internal Medicine
2. Zhang Zhongjing: Treatise on Exogenous Febrile Diseases
3. Ge Hong: Prescriptions for Emergencies
4. Chao Yuanfang: General Treatise on the Causes and Symptoms of Diseases
5. Sun Simiao: Prescriptions Worth a Thousand Gold for Emergencies
6. Chen Shiwen, et al.: Prescriptions of Peaceful Benevolent Despensary
7. Zhang Jingyue: Complete Works of Zhang Jingyue
8. Li Shizhen: Compendium of Materia Medica
9. Wu Qian: The Golden Mirror of Medicine
10. Wu Youxing: Treatise on Pestilence
11. Wang Shixiong: Compendium on Seasonal Febrile Diseases
12. Wu Jutong: Analysis of Epidemic Febrile Diseases
13. Yao Ruoqin, et al.: The Classified Medical Records of Famous Physicians in Song, Yuan, Ming, and Qing Dynasties (1988, 1st edition, Shanghai Bookshop)
14. He Xuan: Teachings on Consumptive Diseases (1984, 1st edition, Shanghai Xuelin Publishing House)
15. Wang Yu: Medical Records beside the Drunken Flower Window (colleted by Shanxi Institute of TCM, 1977)
16. Du Yu Mao: Mechanisms of TCM in the Prophylaxis

and Treatment of AIDS. *Journal of Chengdu TCM College*, 1990; 13 (1): 22.

17. Su Chenglian: Preliminary Personal Experience in the Diagnosis and Treatment of AIDS. *Journal of TCM*, 1990; 2:26.
18. Su Chenglian: Tentative Treatment of AIDS — a clinical report of 30 cases. *Journal of TCM*, 1990; 3:27.
19. Wang Xuao, et al. : Preliminary Approach to Syndrome Differentiation and Therapy Selection of 3 Hemophiliacs Infected by HIV. *Joural of Zhajiang TCM*, 1990; 25 (6): 267.

艾滋病的中医治疗
钟达锦 王绪鳌 赵树珍 傅立宁 编著
王齐亮 译
*
中国山东科学技术出版社出版
（中国济南玉函路）
外文印刷厂印刷
（中国北京车公庄西路）
中国国际图书贸易总公司发行
（中国北京车公庄西路35号）
北京邮政信箱第399号 邮政编码100044
1992年第1版 第1次印刷（英）
ISBN 7-5331-0933-3/R·249（外）
01750
14-E-2652P